"As yoga and mindfulness practices take root in Western soil, they're coming into conversation with the insights and techniques of contemporary psychology. This interaction is modifying both traditions in innumerable ways, and this book is helping to shape that conversation. In different ways, both modern psychology and ancient yoga seek to wake us up from the habits that block us from living lives that matter. This practical book helps us find our footing again."

—**Michael Stone**, author of *The Inner Tradition of Yoga*

"This book offers an enlightening perspective on acceptance and commitment therapy (ACT) using compassion and yoga principles. The exercises are both simple and empowering at the same time, allowing for a deep connection with clients' experiences. This book is the essence of what it means to have an experiential practice."

—**Janina Scarlet, PhD**, clinical psychologist at the Center for Stress and Anxiety Management, author *of Superhero Therapy*, and recipient of the Eleanor Roosevelt Human Rights Award for developing Superhero Therapy

"Yoga plus ACT—how can you possibly ask for a better combination to help you become more flexible as a person? Well, you could ask for such a book to be written by Timothy Gordon and Jessica Borushok. Superb! This book is better than Tantric sex!"

—**D.J. Moran, PhD, BCBA-D**, Pickslyde Consulting

"This is a great book for mental health practitioners, yoga teachers, yoga therapists, and people who want to empower their health on all levels. The content is treated respectfully, and it offers guidelines and tips for people coming at it from various realms of practice. Highly accessible, organized, and at times humorous, the diversity of application and interest makes this a compelling read. There are so many practical, experience-based opportunities to apply the mindful yoga-based acceptance and commitment therapy (MYACT) protocol to improve one's own life, as well as the lives of clients/students!"

—**Erin Byron, MA**, registered psychotherapist, and author of *Yoga for the Creative Soul*

"Whether you are a mental health care or yoga professional, *Mindful Yoga-Based Acceptance and Commitment Therapy* is a unique, balanced blend of wisdom and valuable tools, for and from, both these fields. A great asset as a practical guide in professional trainings or continued education programs, while remaining equally accessible as a step-by-step guide for one's own personal use."

> —**Helene Couvrette, C-IAYT, E-RYT500,** president of MISTY - Montreal International Symposium on Therapeutic Yoga; and founder H~OM Yoga Health Center

"Going way beyond a mere illness model, the authors bring the reader into intimate contact with the science of liberation at the heart of yoga, dharma, and ACT. This is a book for everybody and every body!"

> —**Dennis Tirch**, founder of The Center for Compassion Focused Therapy, associate clinical professor at Mount Sinai, and coauthor of *The ACT Practitioner's Guide to the Science of Compassion*

"This book is immediately accessible and practical for blending yoga and ACT. Doing the work as outlined will bring the reader into a deeply felt understanding of ACT. It's such a brilliant move to blend yoga and ACT, you'll wonder why you didn't think of it. It's also a reader-friendly exploration of the common roots of contextual behavioral science and yoga philosophy and practice."

> —**Joanne Steinwachs, LCSW**, licensed clinical social worker in private practice, and peer-reviewed ACT trainer

"This book is a brilliant contribution not only to the contextual behavioral science literature, but also to the acknowledgement that there are other forms, besides language, to address human struggles. The authors did an incredible job integrating ACT, yoga practices, and a rounded approach to general well-being into a very creative, unique, and step-by-step process. This is certainly a timely book when we have failed to acknowledge the role of our body in our general well-being, and within the field of empirically supported treatments. This book will help all clinicians to expand a repertoire of interventions when working with all clients. A highly recommended book, whether you practice yoga or not!"

> —**Patricia E. Zurita Ona, PsyD**, coauthor of *Mind and Emotions*, and author of *Parenting a Troubled Teen* and *Escaping the Emotional Rollercoaster*

Mindful
YOGA-BASED
Acceptance &
Commitment
Therapy

Simple Postures *and* Practices *to* Help Clients Achieve Emotional Balance

TIMOTHY GORDON, MSW | JESSICA BORUSHOK, PHD
WITH STEVE FERRELL, E-RYT

CONTEXT PRESS
An Imprint of New Harbinger Publications, Inc.

Publisher's Note

This publication is designed to provide accurate and authoritative information in regard to the subject matter covered. It is sold with the understanding that the publisher is not engaged in rendering psychological, financial, legal, or other professional services. If expert assistance or counseling is needed, the services of a competent professional should be sought.

In consideration of evolving American English usage standards, and reflecting a commitment to equity for all genders, "they," "them," and other similar pronouns are used to denote singular persons.

Distributed in Canada by Raincoast Books

Copyright © 2019 by Timothy Gordon, Jessica Borushok, and Steve Ferrell
        Context Press
        An imprint of New Harbinger Publications, Inc.
        5674 Shattuck Avenue
        Oakland, CA 94609
        www.newharbinger.com

Cover design by Amy Shoup

Interior design by Michele Waters-Kermes

Acquired by Elizabeth Hollis-Hansen

Edited by James Lainsbury

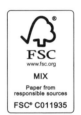 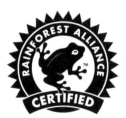

Library of Congress Cataloging-in-Publication Data on file

21   20   19

10   9   8   7   6   5   4   3   2   1   First Printing

For Michael Stone: Yours is a light that will never go out.

—TG, JB, SF

Contents

Introduction

Yoga is an ancient practice more than three thousand years old, and recently it has been the subject of significant empirical research, with good findings, especially for people who suffer from anxiety, stress, chronic pain, or depression. Even people suffering from severe mental health problems, such as schizophrenia, can benefit from this practice. However, health care professionals have been slow to adopt yogic practices, while yoga teachers who want to use yoga to help mental health populations are uncertain of which yogic practices and processes actually work. Adding to the confusion, the yoga community comprises a large range of styles, practices, and even spiritual or theoretical ideas, which makes learning the best practices challenging, to say the least. As a result, there is an understandable distance between the everyday evidence-based best practices of clinical health care professionals and yoga practitioners.

While there is a plethora of empirical support suggesting yoga can benefit mental health issues, researchers have placed little focus on understanding the specific yoga processes and practices that work. For example, research studies rarely distinguish what type of yoga is being looked at or which specific breathing techniques, mindfulness directions, or asanas (structural poses) account for any benefits, let alone do they incorporate mediational analysis to isolate the effective components of yoga. This has led to a cacophony of theories, opinions, and anecdotes about yoga with little grounding in science. And, frankly, this approach is dangerous. Health care professionals and yoga practitioners (us included) have been so excited by the evidence that we forgot to slow down and understand why or what works before rolling out claims that yoga can help those who suffer.

This is where this book—and, more specifically, mindful yoga-based acceptance and commitment therapy/training (or MYACT)—comes in. In it, we will introduce you to the practices of yoga, acceptance and commitment therapy/training (ACT), and the whole health approach to the mind-body connection. You'll learn how to harness yoga's rich wisdom tradition and practices through the lens of modern scientific advances for alleviating suffering. From the perspective that the body and the mind are linked, and that healing psychological suffering requires treating the whole person, MYACT helps therapists and yoga instructors guide clients toward emotional balance and wellness at all levels—physical, psychological, emotional, and spiritual. It does this by melding philosophy with science, and by isolating only the practices that are backed by science, to effectively help those who struggle with painful experiences create a meaningful life.

Yoga teachers and health care professionals are similar in that both arrived at their careers strongly valuing helping others. Both hope to inspire emotional balance and well-ness in clients who are suffering, but problems can arise when these professionals struggle or feel restricted in their abilities to effectively target the turbulent minds of those who suffer with mental health–related problems.

Many people do not respond to talk therapy or seated meditation despite the plethora of documented benefits of these approaches (Eisendrath, Chartier, & McLane, 2011), and movement practices alone, such as those found in yoga classes, are not sufficient to address the emotional and psychological needs of some participants. This book and the protocol within are designed to target these people and present a way to increase *psychological flex-ibility*—that is, the ability to connect with the present and choose how to act based on what's important to that person in that moment, regardless of what painful content shows up. The protocol uses specific evidence-based practices in yoga as an active form of mindfulness in order to train people how to engage these core processes of health and well-being. Health care professionals and yoga teachers alike will come away from this book with a new way to promote emotional balance, valued living, and general wellness in their clients.

MYACT combines the framework of ACT with the core scientifically identified compo-nents of yoga that work to heal. ACT helps people to recognize that trying to avoid or escape painful experiences does not work, and that learning how to accept painful content can help them live a more meaningful, connected life. ACT is already a well-established therapy for increasing psychological flexibility and for helping people achieve emotional balance, both of which it does by encouraging creativity and flexibility. In the case of MYACT, yoga is the tool through which clients are trained in ACT processes, yet it is more than simply learning a few yoga poses. MYACT is understanding how the wisdom and traditions of yoga meld with the science and clarity of ACT to become one. We do not call our protocol "yoga plus ACT" because we view the whole as greater than the sum of its parts.

On its own, yoga provides a physical practice with a rich wisdom tradition that pre-scribes how practitioners should live their lives. And on its own, ACT provides an evidence-based approach to increasing psychological flexibility and well-being, but it is still very much a seated practice of talk therapy. When used together, however, ACT adds context to the prescriptive wisdom traditions of yoga to create more flexibility and autonomy in how one chooses to approach life, suggesting that what matters to each person is unique. Yoga adds techniques and practices (asanas, mantras, meditations) to ACT that can reach those who don't respond to seated meditation or talk therapy or who are interested in a novel, less stigmatized way of healing. Yoga is an experiential way of teaching ACT through movement, helping people connect with and notice sensations in their bodies and any thoughts or feel-ings that arise. The last piece of the MYACT puzzle, whole health, helps us choose, based on who and what matter to us, which behaviors and habits we want to strive for in our efforts to find emotional balance and wellness.

Yoga teachers and health care professionals will both gain wisdom from this book. On one hand, yoga teachers will learn how to use yoga appropriately with mental health populations. They'll learn which practices are evidence based and actually help clients, and which practices to avoid—those that may sound good or are considered "general wisdom" but in reality can be harmful to clients. Yoga teachers will also learn about the principle of psychological flexibility, a measure of emotional balance that may help them deal with emotional or psychological issues that can manifest in class or individual sessions. Health care professionals, on the other hand, will learn how to incorporate yoga practices into their current talk therapy, to use the eight-week MYACT protocol, and to relate to painful cognitive content through the body. They will expand their therapy repertoire with physical relating, and they may be able to reach those who otherwise may not respond to treatment.

About This Book

In this book, we first offer a conceptual understanding of human suffering and provide a strong theoretical foundation for MYACT, followed by three parts. Part 1 covers three distinct subjects: acceptance and commitment therapy/training (ACT), the evidence-based psychological intervention used in MYACT; yoga, including its physical practice and philosophical lineage as organizing principles for ancient teachings and wisdom; and whole health, a modern approach to integrating empirically supported best practices in nutrition, movement, self-care, sleep, and health behavior change. In part 1, we dive deeply into ACT, as epitomized by the ACT matrix and life map. We conclude with an overview of how to safely practice and teach yoga, including information about anatomy and functional movement.

In part 2, we present the MYACT protocol the way we do it, step-by-step, in its most current evolution. Each section in part 2 is a guide for using MYACT in groups. Melding the trifecta of ACT, yoga, and whole health is a large undertaking, which is why we developed the eight-week MYACT protocol. Our hope is that this protocol will provide you with a starting point from which you can weave this practice into yours. The protocol affords plenty of opportunities for creativity and modification along the way so you can make it something uniquely your own that will work with your own client population. We have also made all the worksheets for the program available for download at the website for this book: http://www.newharbinger.com/42358.

Part 3 covers scope of practice considerations for professionals not working in the mental health field. We include information about and skills for implementing this protocol or specific yoga practices in a variety of settings (yoga studio, outpatient groups, inpatient settings) and with individual clients. All health care professionals can incorporate these skills into their practice regardless of whether they have the structural capacity or support to run the full eight-week protocol.

Before You Jump In

Whether you are new to yoga or ACT, or both, this book will provide you with the tools and foundational understanding needed to integrate MYACT into your practice. All information presented in this book is backed by science and informed by the perspectives of a social worker and yoga instructor (Tim), psychologist (Jessica), and yoga instructor (Steve). Our hope is that this book will allow you to view yoga, ACT, and the whole health approach through a unique, unifying lens, revitalizing your personal and professional practice and providing you with the wisdom and knowledge necessary to bring MYACT to your clients and community.

CHAPTER 1

Understanding Human Suffering

This chapter is dedicated to understanding and connecting with the experience of suffering, as it is only through leaning in to our full lived experience, even the painful parts, that we can move forward with a meaningful life. Using the science of acceptance and commitment therapy (ACT) and the wisdom of yoga, we explore how and why people suffer, drawing on the philosophies that support each. In the following journey through the history of the work we do in MYACT we cover a range of topics, from broad foundational ones to specifics of what we choose to do with our pain in any given moment. We finish the journey with a discussion of the whole health model, an approach to living that connects us with the tangible behaviors that move us toward what matters most to us.

Suffering and Psychological Flexibility

ACT therapists and yoga teachers may define suffering differently, but the spirit of healing defines each vocation. And through both personal and professional experience, yoga teachers and ACT therapists understand that all beings on this planet struggle with painful, aversive experiences, and always will. We can no more guarantee the elimination of pain for our clients than we can control when the sun rises each morning.

Suffering, however, emerges as we attempt to avoid, escape, or control painful experiences, rather than sitting with the knowledge that pain is a part of life. The more we fight with ourselves, the harder the struggle becomes and the greater the suffering. A therapist might find herself sitting across from a person who describes a tiny life in which they feel trapped by crippling anxiety. In their desire to not feel pain, the client explains how they no longer drive, go out to see friends, or engage in the activities that once enriched their life with happiness. In a yoga class, a teacher might see a student stay in the back of the class, not attempt more challenging poses, and make self-deprecating comments about not having a "yoga body" due to painful thoughts and memories rather than actual ability in the class. In these situations, suffering comes not from the anxiety one feels, or from the body's inability to bend a certain way, but from the way we try to escape a feeling or sensation we don't like.

If suffering is the result of our attempt to control or avoid pain, rather than the experience of pain itself, then an openness to the truth that pain will always be there and the flexibility to meet that pain and continue forward in our journey are the ways through suffering. When we refuse to come into contact with pain, our world becomes very small and rigid, one focused solely on escape. In ACT, we call this psychological inflexibility, which is the opposite of psychological flexibility, our model of healing and emotional balance.

We define *psychological inflexibility* as attempts to avoid, control, or escape a painful experience that limit one's repertoire (what one does when pain shows up) and negatively impact long-term quality of life. Psychological inflexibility is about what someone does in a specific situation and how well that behavior works. An ACT therapist is interested in the things people do to try and limit their contact with the thoughts, feelings, sensations, and memories they don't want, and to understand how their attempts to limit that contact may also be impacting their connection to what matters most in life. It is normal to try to protect ourselves from pain and perceived threats. However, attempts to escape, avoid, or control painful experiences become problematic when they interfere with a life well lived (for example, avoiding relationships or intimacy for fear of rejection, working long hours to escape downtime when upsetting thoughts pop up). Note that this definition does not suggest that escaping, avoiding, or attempting to control painful experiences is purely pathological. Sometimes avoidance is helpful! Our focus is on understanding which behaviors don't move people toward the life they want to live, whatever that may be.

A person suffering from anxiety may not be able to overtly explain to you their psychological inflexibility, but if you listen closely and watch what happens when anxiety shows up in the form of panic attacks, worrisome thoughts, self-reported heart pounding, or sweating, you'll see psychological inflexibility in their attempts to escape what they don't want to feel. This presentation may look different for different people. One person may stop driving in response to fear or a panic attack. In response to thoughts that they have to keep up to avoid looking foolish, others might force themselves deeper into yoga postures than is safe in an attempt to mimic what they see around them in the studio rather than using the feedback from their body to guide their practice. Another person might avoid social situations or places, or stay in a job that they hate, rather than trying something new or chasing a more meaningful life. When it comes to psychological inflexibility, the point is not what we see people doing but how what they're doing works in their situation.

Remember, the goal is not to remove pain. The goal is to halt unworkable attempts to escape or avoid pain that lead to suffering, to be flexible rather than rigid in the presence of pain. Yoga and ACT perceive pain similarly: not as a disease to be cured but a source of information. Physical pain informs yoga practitioners. It tells them to be gentle and to listen to their body, to notice how muscle groups compensate, to be cautious, and to be aware of how the nervous system communicates through breath and sensation. Emotional or cognitive pain informs ACT practitioners. Painful mental content (thoughts, feelings, memories, physical sensations) is related to something important, so they know to listen closely to this pain in order to understand what matters.

Humans have a unique ability to bring pain into awareness, even when painful experiences are not present. A wolf may be cold and hungry, but as soon as it has food in its belly and it is curled up and warm in a cave with other wolves, the wolf does not think about its next meal. But a warm, safe, and satiated human can ruminate on where the next meal might come from. This last point is extremely important: humans have a unique ability to experience pain, even when they are not directly presented with it. Through thoughts and memories we can bring painful experiences into any moment and dream up potential future problems. This ability can cause unlimited suffering, and it can take people out of the moment they are actually living. Advances in behavioral science explain why.

Relational Frame Theory (RFT) and Yogic Sādhanā

Relational frame theory (RFT) is a scientific, empirically supported theory that posits that language, the things we think and feel, is a behavior, and that this behavior occurs within a relational network of thoughts, feelings, memories, physical sensations, and experiences. It further suggests that this relational network can be linked to others, thereby creating complex connections between experiences that may not seem obvious or apparent. This ability to create relational networks and complex connections between experiences is what allows us to create symbolic meaning for objects. For example, it's how a piece of paper becomes valuable through its representation as currency. It's also what allows us to connect places, objects, and people with thoughts about future worst-case scenarios, trauma memories, and labels about our abilities or the roles we have. It's how worry about a future meal can show up when we're safe, well fed, and warm.

Once these networks and connections are made, they cannot be removed; we cannot unlearn or erase a painful memory or upsetting thought. The only option is to make more connections. This is important to understand: although people may attempt to avoid, control, or escape their most painful private experiences, that pain is permanently inescapable. There is no delete button for what shows up inside of us. No matter how hard we try, we can never permanently remove or delete painful experiences from our relational networks— they are a part of our experience, and we can no more stop a painful thought from popping up than we can stop the sensation of physical pain when we break a leg.

When we begin to recognize the unworkability of attempts to avoid, escape, or delete painful content, we can change our focus, or create flexibility, in the presence of this pain and the networks it creates.

One way we can create flexibility is to see ourselves as being separate from our experiences. We are the observers of all these connections and experiences. For example, there is a you behind your eyes reading the words on this page, taking in the information, and working through what it means in the form of thoughts in your mind. By understanding the impact this has on our life, and by noticing our drive to escape or avoid, we can instead choose to behave in a different way. Rather than reacting automatically, unsuccessfully running away from pain, we can choose to behave in ways that move us closer to what matters in life. Freedom lies in having the ability to choose what we do no matter what pain our mind brings into the present.

Of course, RFT was not the first theory to bring forth this idea. Far from it. More than 2,500 years ago, the Indian sage Patañjali (or potentially a group of teachers producing a document under one name) published the Yoga Sūtras, a collection of poetic yoga wisdom writings inspired by early Mahayana Buddhism, the eight limbs of yoga, and action yoga in an attempt to answer the question of why humans suffer and how to address this suffering. In Yoga Sūtra 1.3, Patañjali writes, "*tadā draṣṭuḥ svarūpe-'vasthānam*," which most accurately translates to "Then [through yoga] the Seer abides in Itself" (Āranya, 1984, 11; Remski, 2012, 46). This verse has also been translated more poetically as "for finding our true self (drashtu) entails insight into our own nature" (AYI, n.d.). A more technical translation is "When thought ceases, the spirit stands in its true identity as observer to the world" (Miller, 1998, 29).

Many other interpretations of this passage exist, with inferences to the meaning of the passage, but we feel Miller's (1998) treatment—"the spirit stands in its true identity as observer to the world"—most relevantly captures Patañjali's answer: to unjoin the transcendent self and the content of one's experience. Simply put, the path through suffering is to be the observer of one's experience. Up until Patañjali's writing, the reigning idea in Buddhist tradition had been that there was no self, rather everything was one. So Patañjali's perspective was fresh for its time, and, as we see in RFT today, it's still relevant.

Such a feat of awareness, as described by Patañjali, is now an essential component of increasing psychological flexibility. This perspective, to be the observer of our experience— that there is a self behind our eyes that sees our thoughts, feelings, memories, sensations— allows us to take a step back from our painful experiences and notice how we react to them, what we do when they show up, and whether that behavior takes us closer to the life we want to live. In this space between ourselves and our experience lies our ability to choose how we want to behave, rather than being sucked into emotion or stuck to a thought or rule that governs our behavior.

Said more explicitly, Patañjali's goal to separate the seer from all thought and experience is the same as ACT's goal to separate the self from the content of one's life, including thoughts, feelings, sensations, memories, roles, and so forth. *Self-as-content* is the term ACT uses to describe becoming fused with the labels, qualities, and roles that we ascribe to our self and that can interfere with our ability to be psychologically flexible. Both ACT and yoga maintain that this place—in the private experience of the self that we each endure—is where suffering happens. Our experiences teach us lessons about who we think we are. Our layers of experiencing, relating, and acting are learned behaviors with outcomes that shape what we do next.

If we, for instance, have a history of failed relationships, we may begin to find fault with ourselves or think *I am unlovable*. If we hold this belief tightly and are unable to step back from the painful content, it may influence whether we put effort into connecting with others in the future. And over time, with repetition and exposure, this learning constructs habitual patterns—what in yogic scholarship are called samskāras. This verse, from the Yoga Sūtras, encapsulates this idea: "Fruitlessly seeking consolation, alienating patterns of thought tend to repeat. This repetition can impede self-perception, relationship to time, and the capacity for enjoyment. Alienating patterns predispose you to continued alienation" (Remski, 2012, 32). Since premedieval times, Eastern wisdom has espoused that beliefs about who we are, what we can or can't do, and what we do or don't deserve cause us pain. They also dictate actions that further our suffering.

In yoga, Patañjali challenges us to look deeply into the way we frame ourselves in relation to our experience and the world around us. Patañjali posits that living unaware is failing to learn how to change thoughts, ideas, sensations, and self-content (Remski, 2012). Similarly, RFT helps us understand how we frame ourselves through language, including our private behavior of thinking, feeling, sensing, and remembering, and the connections that our thoughts, feelings, sensations, and memories share. To transform suffering, to go from living on autopilot to noticing each moment, we must develop the ability to observe this mental content and understand how it can become related to the self.

In ACT, we harness two other perspectives of the self to do this. One is *self-as-process*, an awareness of the ongoing stream of experiencing—thinking, feeling, sensing, remembering, behaving. Yoga can be an incredible tool for experiencing such an awareness. In yoga, you inhabit self-as-process every time you connect with moment-to-moment changes in sensations or other mental content as you move from one pose in a sequence to another. The other perspective ACT employs is *self-as-context*, an understanding of the self as being distinct from one's experience, and the corresponding ability to shift awareness from behind our eyes to behind the eyes of another (see the world from another's perspective), or to view the world from behind our eyes at a different point in time (see the world from the perspective of our younger self or future self). The self-as-context is the self Patañjali refers to when he writes about the seer abiding in itself. It is a self or soul that can be liberated from the changing states of one's mind.

Once we develop such an understanding of the self and cultivate the practice of stepping back from the content of our mind, we can choose how we respond to that content and how we live our life and connect with what matters to us. In MYACT, we refer to what matters as *values*, the who and what that matter to you, the qualities or characteristics you want to be about, and your "true north" that you are continuously striving to reach.

So the goal in ACT, and in MYACT, has two prongs: First, we strive to free clients from the psychological inflexibility produced by self-as-content, which limits them to rigid rules that might only allow them to attempt to escape, avoid, or control painful experiences, no matter the context or situation. Second, we introduce flexibility to their actions, so they can choose how to behave based on the specific situation they find themselves in, and so they can choose to work toward their values regardless of the pain that shows up.

Yoga provides us the opportunity to connect with our mental and physical content through movement practices. The experience of coming into contact with painful content can be intense, and as a result, yoga can seem like a safe introduction to this practice of noticing, as physical sensations are generally easier for most people to notice than the mental content of thoughts and feelings. While we do contact the mental content in yoga practice, we begin from a place of noticing how the body moves, because doing so helps to train each person to tune in to their experience. Later on, we work to expand that noticing to one's full experience.

In our introduction, we mentioned how yoga has wisdom traditions that essentially pre-scribe how a person should live life. Patañjali's Yoga Sūtras describe seven stages divided into eight limbs, popularly referred to as the steps toward the final stage of *samādhi*, or enlightenment. The function, therefore, of Patañjali's Yoga Sūtras was to not only acknowl-edge the perspective of the self as the observer of the world, but to also escape the experi-ence of struggling and pass into a world, or state, called enlightenment. We do not seek enlightenment in MYACT, rather we use this perspective and that of RFT to enhance how our clients live in and interact with this world. The following section explores Tantrik philosophy and functional contextualism, providing insight and tools for how to live more fully in this life from the perspective of the observer.

Functional Contextualism and Tantrik Philosophy

Assessing the flexibility of one's psychology is part of a scientific movement called func-tional contextualism—"function" meaning what works, and "context" meaning in a certain situation. Avoiding, escaping, or attempting to control a painful experience is often unhelp-ful. But in particular contexts, such behaviors might work (function) in a way that *is* in fact helpful. To know which is the case, we have to look at the function of a behavior rather than just the behavior itself. This too is the ultimate aim in ACT: to help clients understand the function of behaviors in a specific context, and with that knowledge, work to decrease unworkable behaviors and increase workable behaviors—those that bring people closer to the life they want to live, or their values.

While functional contextualism focuses on each specific moment, the yogic philosophy of Tantra focuses on how to live life as a whole, consistently embracing the conditions of one's life as a way to meet the world more fully. Whereas Patañjali's Yoga Sūtras (written between 500 BCE and 200 CE) show us how to interact with our painful content, Tantra (developed between 350 and 500 CE) shows us how we might interact with the world. Tantra concerns itself not with escaping suffering or finding an altered state in enlightenment, but rather with how we can engage with the world and the pain we have to reach a meaningful life. It is a terrific complement to functional contextualism. Together, these philosophies teach us how to come into contact with pain we experience and to understand the function of our behaviors so we may chase our values in life.

Tantrik philosophy also informs *asana*, the physical practice of yoga in our MYACT protocol. In Tantra, asana is viewed as an opportunity to meet the changes of the body, a metaphor for the way Tantra also informs living in the world. Historically, Tantrik practices encouraged *svādhyāya*, or "self study," in order to bring about a deeper connection to what we hold most valuable (Stephens, 2010), suggesting we do this through yoga asana, meditation, chanting, and breath work. We incorporate these same strategies in MYACT.

The expectations of postures, alignment, form, and ability in yoga are not fixed but instead contextually informed (based on what is happening in that moment). So, from a practical standpoint, the way yoga is instructed encourages practitioners to meet their body where it is in the moment—that is, to be flexible. Therefore, in our instruction of yoga asana we may ask questions to inspire this Tantrik perspective: What kind of body are you working with today? What kind of strength is meeting your practice today? What expectations do you have of your flexibility today? What kind of mind are you working with today? Every day, and for every practice and every asana, our body and mind are different. If we are sensitive to that difference, if we get at the specific function a movement has in the context of our practice, we can adjust and flexibly meet each posture, ensuring that our movements work to bring us closer to what is important to us in that moment (values, showing our body kindness).

And this perspective on life extends off the mat. We encourage clients to move through their day with a sensitivity to what may be different, to take the present-moment awareness into everyday living. Tantra encourages people to notice the changes in contextual factors so as to better understand the function of their behavior (Feuerstein, 2008; Stephens, 2010). Again, this broader perspective on how to live life and meet the world blends beautifully with functional contextualism's focus on how actions work to take us closer to or further from our values in each unique moment.

An important aspect of this perspective lies in the way we view truth. Within functional contextualism, truth is assessed through function—what works and what doesn't. Functional contextualists don't concern themselves with capital T truths, rather they focus on function and work to understand what maintains certain behaviors that aren't functional in relation to the long-term goal of vitality.

For example, imagine a person who wholeheartedly identifies, or is fused, with the thought *I am fat and ugly*. Every time that thought shows up, this person experiences pain in the form of sadness and anger and despair. In order to make those feelings go away, the individual eats sweets despite having the value of living a healthy lifestyle. For functional contextualists, it does not matter whether this painful thought is the capital T truth. This person may be "ugly" or "fat" by societal and medical standards, or not. It is not the truth of the matter that causes the person's suffering. Rather, it is this person's efforts to appease or dampen the painful feelings related to that thought, through excessive eating, that cause suffering. The suffering is the pattern of painful thought, painful feeling, and brief relief from pain while eating, followed by increased suffering. Not only does this person still think the same things and feel the same way, but now they feel shame for what they ate and have self-reprimanding thoughts about their behavior. In this instance, a functional contextualist would focus on how eating in the short term is reinforcing and provides temporary relief, but in the long term, attempting to eliminate painful thoughts and feelings only increases suffering and keeps this person further from the life they want to lead.

With this understanding of truth in mind, our goal in MYACT is to use this functional contextualism analysis to target suffering with helpful interventions that increase a person's ability to look at and understand the function of behavior in different contexts and choose new, more adaptive behaviors. This is in contrast to focusing on the form of a behavior, what it looks like, and judging it to be wrong, bad, or maladaptive based on personal, cultural, or philosophical stances. Functional contextualism doesn't prescribe a "right" way of being or living in the world, and Tantra invites one to embrace the painful content of life as a way to meet the world more fully, whatever that may look like to the individual. Yoga (informed by Tantra) and ACT (informed by functional contextualism) together in this MYACT protocol are about facing the challenges of living, whatever they may be, with flexibility. This is done with both a broader long-term perspective of meeting the world and an in-the-moment evaluation of function in the service of living a meaningful life.

The truth is that most of us these days do not meet the world fully. Often we settle into patterns of similarity or avoidance, making it easier to approach life from a place of automaticity, or on autopilot. When we stop paying attention to the pain in our lives and the experiences around us, we become insensitive to context. This insensitivity is pathological in our functional contextual viewpoint because it leads to a pattern of reacting in order to escape unpleasant experiences regardless of what is happening in that moment or what is important to the person. We stop showing up to each moment and making a choice of how we want to live in each moment.

In MYACT, we train clients how to notice what is occurring in the present moment. This training happens through yoga poses, breath work, engagement with the life map, and at-home practices. But the goal is always the same: to help people connect more fully with their full experience so that they can better evaluate whether how they are living is working for them and can see opportunities to do something differently. This is not something we can do for them. Only they can decide if how they are living works for them. We integrate this in our teachings in MYACT via an Eastern philosophical sentiment we subscribe to, that each person must walk their own path. As we say to participants early in MYACT, "No one can do this practice for you." However, MYACT provides participants the context and tools with which to evaluate whether their life is working for them, and if not, which changes may need to happen to live a meaningful life.

So, Patañjali and relational frame theory help us understand why people suffer; Tantrik philosophy, through yoga, meditation, breathing, and chanting, teaches us to focus our attention on connecting more fully with the life we are living now; and functional contextualism provides us the truth criterion of function to evaluate how we are living and interacting with our suffering in a specific moment or context. We cultivate MYACT participants' awareness of all of this using yoga and ACT, and we guide them to slow down and find a space in which to choose to change their habits or actions in that moment. And how does this habit change work? The final piece of MYACT's foundation, whole health, provides the tangible skills and direction for making lasting behavior change.

Whole Health

The more we notice and evaluate our behavior, the more options for how we live our life will emerge. Whole health encourages meaningful, long-term behavior change while providing a foundation of skills and common meaningful domains to increase the likelihood of values-based actions in those moments of choice. In MYACT, we provide multiple examples of aspects of life—nutrition, sleep, habit change, movement, interacting with others—that contribute to well-being and emotional balance, transforming the abstract concept of values into concrete, tangible, committed actions. Through in-the-moment practice, we create the context through which participants can transform behaviors, moving beyond traditional strategies of psychoeducation, or beyond simply telling people what is good for them. We link what we do in the yoga studio or therapy room with how we live our life outside of that moment. And really, this is what whole health is all about: applying evidence-based strategies to aspects of our lives that can enhance our health in multiple domains (physical, emotional, spiritual) and increase our ability to move in a valued direction because whole health itself creates a strong foundation from which to explore our context.

We chose to incorporate whole health components into our MYACT protocol for two reasons: they often create meaning in one's life, but they can also cause suffering when there is confusion or lack of movement. Focusing on creating a healthy lifestyle—beyond simply sleeping more, eating vegetables, and landing a cool-looking yoga pose—can transform a person's life, adding vitality and a richness in meaning. A mountain of evidence backs this up. It is the process of continuously striving that inspires change, and whole health can inform the small steps that can keep us moving forward. Consider the person who identifies connecting with loved ones as a value but struggles to figure out what that looks like in practice. Or the person who values being a hard worker but struggles to focus at work due to sleep difficulties. For both people, specific whole health information or techniques can help them move toward their value, whereas otherwise they may remain stuck, with intention but no direction. Simply practicing mindfulness daily or incorporating a brief yoga pose into an evening routine can be a struggle to sort out, and whole health components can provide structure, information, and skills to make building new habits more successful.

Whole health represents the little actions we incorporate into our day-to-day life to make the work we do in each MYACT session most effective and impactful. We encourage participants to take the work done in group outside into their own life and provide both practices of the mind and body to set them on a path toward a life of meaning, whatever that means to them. MYACT helps people set an intention to change, develops behaviors to support this change, and provides guidance—backed by science—to ensure they are moving toward a life of whole health, as outlined by their personal values.

Bringing It All Together

ACT and yogic philosophy set the stage for the stance, or perspective, we bring to our practice of MYACT. With each pose or exercise, we take participants from the philosophy of life to the doing of living. Yoga encourages strength, stability, and flexibility (all important aspects of exercise). It enhances awareness of the body and how it functions, a perspective that advocates for doing kinder things to our body (sleep, recovery) and for adding vibrant fuel to it (whole foods). Yoga encourages practitioners to interact with others from this same position of kindness and compassion, deeper intimacy, compromise, and flexibility. ACT of course only bolsters and provides a framework from which to understand processes we may already be doing, or processes that are naturally occurring but one cannot name, intentionally replicate, or teach. It provides tools and creates purpose so that how we live our life, who we interact with, and what we say and do is intentional and focused on what matters most to us. Both the practice of yoga and the model of ACT work on their own to promote wellness and an integrated picture of vitality. They both inherently promote whole health, so it's not surprising that they complement each other so well. And together, they create MYACT.

Now that you understand the three schools of thinking that inform MYACT (ACT, yoga, whole health), and why this book is bringing them together—to help clients become more flexible in the presence of their pain in order to live a life of meaning—we're ready to move deeper into specifics.

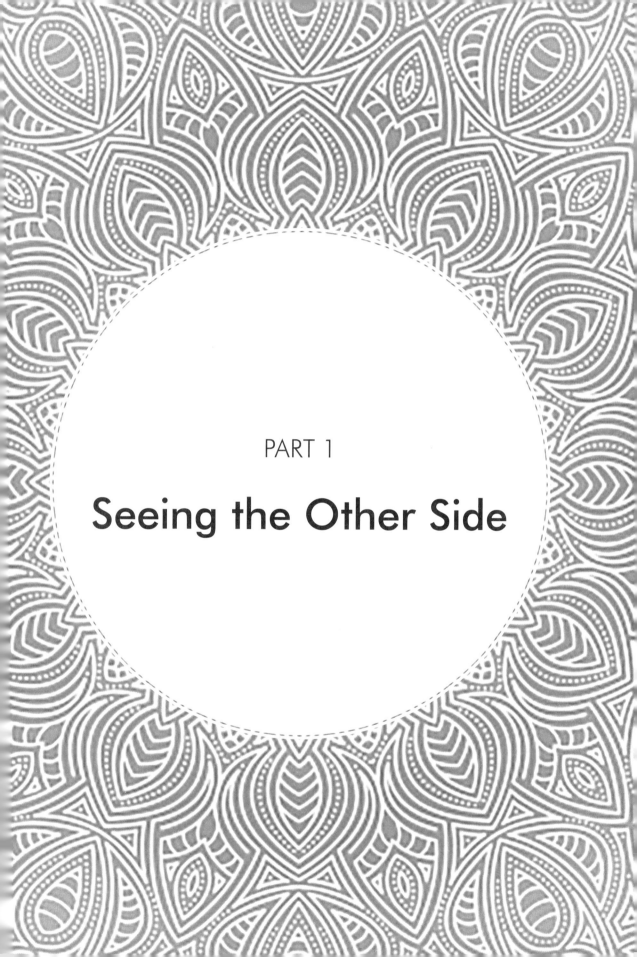

PART 1

Seeing the Other Side

There is a wealth of information related to the disciplines of yoga, ACT, and the whole health approach to living. Our goal with this book is not to exhaust your attention with an in-depth discussion of each, but rather to tell a story of how the principles, lessons, and philosophies of these disciplines coalesce such that the resulting product—MYACT—is greater than the sum of its parts. Our ultimate goal is to provide therapists and yoga instructors with better tools for working with people who are suffering, and we feel that a good starting place is to educate you both about the other's discipline. Thus, the following two chapters are dedicated to providing a deeper understanding of each. Yoga teachers will learn more about ACT and a tool called the life map, while mental health professionals will explore anatomy and ways to cue functional movement in participants. This first part of the book will set the foundation for the MYACT protocol, described in part 2.

CHAPTER 2

ACT Through the Life Map

In this book, we've described both yoga and ACT academically, positing that yoga ought to be experienced as a model for being and ACT a model for living. In this chapter, rather than explaining to you how ACT works, we elected to *show* you. This book, after all, is about experience. It's one thing to describe the colors of a sunset and quite another to see that sunset. In this vein, we're going to invite you to experience ACT.

To assist us in doing so, we adapted the ACT matrix created by Kevin Polk, Jerold Hambright, and Mark Webster (Polk, 2014). The ACT matrix is a tool for helping clients observe their patterns of behavior and for training them to better evaluate a pattern's function and to increase their engagement with actions tied to a meaningful life. We call this adaptation the life map (Gordon & Borushok, 2017), and it's just that: a map of what you experience both in the observable world and privately (sensations, feelings, thoughts, and emotions). The life map allows participants the opportunity to take a step back, get some perspective on how their patterns of behavior work for them, and identify what their next steps are based on where they most wish to go. Below, we will walk you through setting up the life map and have you answer specific questions to teach you noticing skills and to identify how functional (or how workable) your current patterns of behavior are.

Through the life map, we will introduce you to the six independent yet connected core processes of psychological flexibility that make up the work we do in ACT: values, defusion, acceptance, commitment, present moment, and self-as-context. The life map is a primary tool of the eight-week protocol, so it will be helpful for you to see how the six core processes relate to it. As we guide you through the life map, we'll give you all the tools you need to understand and use ACT.

The Life Map

To begin your very own life map, draw a horizontal line with arrowheads at each end. At the center, draw a star and write "You are here." The arrowheads depict moving in different directions. The right side is about chasing values, and the left is about escaping pain.

Situating yourself in the middle of the map, just like you would see in a directory at a shopping mall, is about you being the observer of your experience, the author of your values who is separate from your pain, the witness to what is difficult for you. Being at the center of your map is about being more aware of how what you're doing works, so that you can more easily choose what you want your life to be about.

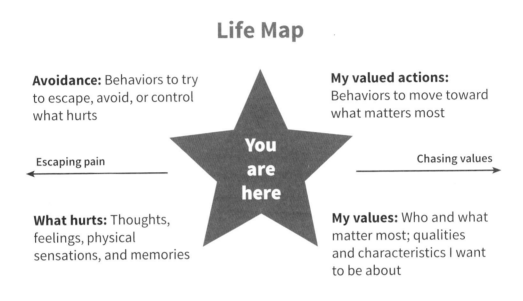

Life Map

Avoidance: Behaviors to try to escape, avoid, or control what hurts

My valued actions: Behaviors to move toward what matters most

Escaping pain ←

→ Chasing values

You are here

What hurts: Thoughts, feelings, physical sensations, and memories

My values: Who and what matter most; qualities and characteristics I want to be about

Adapted from Gordon & Borushok (2017)

The life map is divided into four quadrants, each one meant to track different types of information. In the bottom right, we pose a simple question: Who and what are most important to you? This is a values-based question focused on the long-term distal reinforcers (things that are reinforcing in the long term) that are uniquely important to each person. Take a moment and reflect on who and what matter most to you. Think of the people who are important in your life now, the people who have mattered, the people who you want to build a new connection with. When asking yourself what is important, you might be tempted to write something specific, like money. If so, pause and ask why that matters to you. Perhaps financial independence is uniquely important to you. What would more money afford you in your life? Similarly, if you answered happiness, that's great, because happiness is wonderful, but what is that about for you? We're looking for deeper meaning about what is important. If you were happy, what would your life look like? What would change? More broadly, you can also list the qualities you want to be about in your pursuit of connecting with who and what matter most. For each of us writing this book, we could say we value writing a great book, but there's something deeper there for each of us: spreading evidence-based information, sharing innovations and encouraging growth, having fun with a new project!

Values

Helping participants make explicit who and what are most important to them and what they most wish to be about is the values-focused work in MYACT that guides where they want to go in life. This values authorship clarifies what might be different, a new direction they might take in the presence of pain.

The bottom-left quadrant is for listing the painful private experiences (thoughts, feelings, physical sensations, and memories) that get in the way of you chasing your values. These are the thoughts, feelings, sensations, or memories that you struggle with. Take special care not to list difficult situations or people. If there's someone or something external in your life that's hard for you, ask yourself what makes it difficult for you. What thoughts, judgments, evaluations, or painful feelings show up about this? Problems arise when we become fused with these private experiences, when we begin to hear a thought or judgment as fact and become overwhelmed with our fears. One goal of MYACT is to make space for or to defuse from this painful content.

Defusion

Being able to recognize all private content as just that, material in the ongoing flow of private experiences (thoughts, feelings, sensations, and memories), encourages participants to pay attention to these experiences and to track the potential impact of taking them literally.

As we move out of the world of private behavior, we turn our attention to the observable things we do. The top-left quadrant is for tracking what you do to avoid, control, and escape painful experiences. Essentially, this quadrant is for listing what happens when you buy into and believe to be true all the painful private experiences you listed in the bottom-left quadrant. Reflect on the difficult things that show up in the bottom-left quadrant. What do you do to avoid, control, and escape these things? Write down any behaviors you come up with. Try not to judge them as good or bad or to force yourself to make a list of strictly pathological behaviors.

In functional contextualism, there's no such thing as maladaptive behavior. All behavior has a function. For example, maybe you go for a run to try to make feelings of anger go away. Your challenge is to simply notice how you react to painful content when you try to get away from it, if only for a moment. This tracking can be tricky, because some of what we do seems helpful. Things like planning, thinking through "what if" scenarios, and running through upsetting past memories to come up with a solution may feel helpful, but if you slow down and look at the behavior's function, you may find that often it's just another way to avoid pain!

Acceptance

Accepting one's experience is about engaging with painful private experiences (thoughts, feelings, sensations, memories) without restriction. It is normal to try and escape something you do not want to feel. Acceptance is about being sensitive to when attempts to escape are not workable—when they fail to permanently delete painful content or keep us from moving closer to what we value—and instead leaning into pain so we can take a step in a valued direction. This is part of ending the cycle of avoidance and escape. As we've said before, life involves pain, and acknowledging this fact, allowing pain to be a part of life, keeps us from running in circles, exhausting ourselves trying to never feel pain.

Once you have a list of behaviors (two or three will do) in the top-left quadrant, we can move on to the top-right quadrant, which is for listing behaviors that you could do or that you're already doing to chase your values. What you list here is different from the bottom-right quadrant, where you listed values. These are behaviors that drive you closer to your values—things you can be seen doing, that can be ticked off a list, that you're already doing or want to be doing. If you wrote "be happy," try taking it a step further, as being happy is not an observable behavior. For example, if we could watch you live your life (in a noncreepy way) and move toward what matters to you, what would we see you do? If the temptation to write "not eat donuts" or "not argue" arises, focus on what you would be doing instead, such as eating kale, or saying "I love you" to your spouse. What would you want to commit to that takes you closer to your values? Sometimes it's helpful to start small. What is one thing you could do each day to move closer to your values?

Commitment

Commitment is about behavior change, doing new things, persisting, or staying the course in a difficult situation. Acting upon one's values or simply practicing the other four core processes of psychological flexibility could alone represent commitment. In MYACT, one of our favorite ways to play with the concept of commitment is to notice how a particular behavior is working during yoga practice. In one situation, dropping to one's knees and resting in Child's Pose during a vigorous yoga practice might be a commitment to self-care and being gentle with one's body, whereas at a different time, this same behavior could be about escaping an uncomfortable judgment that shows up with shortness of breath: *I'm not fit like the other participants. I should quit. This is embarrassing.*

It's really up to participants to pay careful attention and to assess the function of their behavior, but using the language of commitment makes explicit our behavior-change agenda and gives us a common language. Again, commitment is not about good or bad behaviors. It's about what takes us closer to the life we want to live. As alluded to with the example above, the same behavior can function in two different ways: one to connect with values and the other to escape pain.

Take a step back and look at the life map you've created. This is a map to your life. You stated who and what matter most to you, you noticed the pain that shows up in your life that can make it hard to engage in a life that matters, you tracked your behaviors to escape that pain, and you uncovered what you do to chase your values. Take a moment to notice what it feels like to chase your values. For some people it's exciting, or perhaps just natural, whereas for others it might feel risky or effortful. What is it like for you? Remember, this work is all about noticing, so there is no wrong answer.

Let's now contrast what it feels like to chase your values with what it feels like to try to escape, avoid, or control painful inner experiences. Many people tell us the latter feels good in the short term, perhaps tinged of guilt. Like popping a pimple or itching a mosquito bite, the action works in the moment but is regretted later. Others say it's just downright terrible. Some people spend so much time attempting to escape that it just feels normal. If judgments show up for you while thinking about this, try not to get too caught up in your own evaluation of these experiences. Instead, stick to the task of noticing what each judgment feels like.

Present Moment

Orienting oneself to any experience that may be occurring here and now—shifting awareness to pay attention to and notice the ongoing flow of thoughts, feelings, memories, and sensory experiences—is a crucial yet distinct process in ACT's approach to health. The more we cultivate the practice of noticing what is happening in the present moment, the better we are at evaluating the function of our behaviors and the more freedom we have to choose what we do in any particular moment.

Your life map shows the entirety of your experience, but it wouldn't be complete without something that represents where you fit into your experience. That is why at the center of the map is a star; that star is you. You are the observer of everything that happens in your life.

Self-as-Context

Separating private content (the things we think, feel, sense, and remember) from the one who observes the content (one's consciousness) is situating the self as the context of the experience: the observer self. Patañjali postulated that people who solely identify with their self-as-content (when one is fused with thoughts, judgments, stories, or roles) have bound themselves to a nonpermanent reality that causes suffering. ACT similarly conceptualizes this fusion with self-content as potentially problematic. We say "potentially" because there are times when fusion with self-content can be helpful or useful. For example, thinking *I am a caring therapist* or *I'm a thoughtful yoga instructor* can be beneficial if fusing with either role encourages you to continue learning and striving to find new ways to help clients. Remember, the key to figuring out whether something is problematic or useful is to come back to the core philosophical position of workability: is fusion with self-content in this particular situation effective? In general, though, we want to train ourselves to notice our experience so we are in a better position to intentionally choose how we want to behave next.

Making Life Maps

Now that you've experienced the life map for yourself, let's take a step back and look at what we did in that exercise so you understand the ins and outs of the process and can re-create it with ease with participants in the eight-week protocol. We asked you a series of questions and gave some careful direction. The questions are meant to elicit specific information. When we asked who and what are most important to you, we were looking for values, the distal reinforcers that are not simply obtained and completed. To make this more concrete, imagine that you wrote that your intimate relationship with your partner is important to you. You can't simply wake up, smile at your partner, offer a compliment, wish them a good day, and then cross "intimate relationship" off your list. Values are a process, not a goal with an ending. Said more simply, you can't place a checkmark next to these behaviors and consider them done. They may be relevant on a particular day, but many more behaviors continue after them, all organized and driven by a value, such as your intimate relationship.

When creating the life map, we assessed for (1) values, (2) fused private content, (3) avoidance and escape behaviors, (4) and committed actions, and then we (5) took a step back and tracked what it's like to move toward our values and to attempt to escape painful experiences. Let's expand on the last step to look at the short-term and long-term impacts of chasing values and escaping pain.

Often, when people escape or avoid a painful feeling or thoughts, they experience an immediate sense of relief, even if just for a single moment. This makes avoidance incredibly reinforcing. Whenever we avoid, we remove something unpleasant—that is, pain. However, when we decide to avoid at the cost of not chasing our values, this behavior has long-term consequences. Maybe we experience guilt, or that pain we wanted to escape comes back even stronger.

The inverse is usually true of moving toward what matters to us, of chasing our values. Initially, taking a step toward our values and engaging in a committed action is scary. Maybe it involves having a difficult conversation or setting boundaries, maybe it increases your fear or anxiety in the short term, or maybe it feels unsafe. It's a misconception that values-based actions are easy and feel good. Often, they feel quite the opposite. However, over time, the long-term impact of stepping toward values increases one's quality of life. While it may not be easy, it is immensely comforting to know you are living a life that is in line with everything you care most about. Besides, the hardest things in life are often those that are most worth the effort. Cheesy, we know, but true nonetheless.

This process of looking at the short-term and long-term impacts of behaviors is the crux of assessing their function. Asking clients to notice whether their behavior is intended to help them avoid something and achieve short-term relief or to embody their values, which is harder but opens the door for real change, allows us to highlight the long-term costs of continued avoidance and to point out that it doesn't actually work. One cannot escape pain. By looking at their own experience as the observer, they can begin to recognize patterns. When they slow down and make space to see both their private and observable behaviors, they can better evaluate their function and recognize that, in the long term, avoidance doesn't actually remove painful experiences. Not only that, it can increase suffering and take them farther from the values-driven life they want to live. This perspective can often give people the courage to try something else, and to be willing to experience or lean into pain in order to better connect with values.

Five Questions to Set Up the Life Map

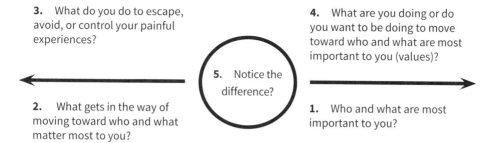

3. What do you do to escape, avoid, or control your painful experiences?

4. What are you doing or do you want to be doing to move toward who and what are most important to you (values)?

5. Notice the difference?

2. What gets in the way of moving toward who and what matter most to you?

1. Who and what are most important to you?

Adapted from Gordon & Borushok (2017)

Knowing the Landscape

Over time, we have come to reference the life map throughout the MYACT protocol, especially when working with individual clients. We find ourselves returning to it again and again, not just as a common language for talking about the contrast between chasing values or attempting to avoid pain but also as a point of reference, like how you might open a map of familiar territory to become reacquainted with some fine detail or to reorient yourself. The life map offers you opportunities to pause and reflect on experiences, looking at where you've been and where you want to go while maintaining a consistent perspective as the observer. With the life map, we can teach participants how to use ACT's six core processes to increase psychological flexibility.

Before you begin a MYACT group or session, we encourage you to make a life map for yourself or with a friend, neighbor, someone you love, a client, or a community group. The more experience you have using the life map with different people and different problems, the better you will be at pinpointing how patterns of behavior function, regardless of what words are used to describe a particular issue.

We hope this chapter informed those readers completely unfamiliar with ACT and provided clarification and review for those who are familiar with it. In the next chapter, we move from the mind to the body. It includes information necessary to be an effective MYACT facilitator and to teach yoga from a functional perspective.

CHAPTER 3

What You Need to Know to Teach Yoga

In this chapter, we cover what you need to know about anatomy, posture, breathing techniques, and functional movement in order to teach and practice yoga. We begin by discussing how we conceptualize and teach others about mindfulness and the breath, as our perspective and methods may differ from those you've encountered. We then explore the skeletal system and how the body can move. We end by offering language, or cues, you can use to draw participants' attention to how they are moving and what adjustments they can make.

The Breath and Mindfulness

MYACT uses mindfulness as a noticing and comprehensive distancing technique, defined as a way for people to defuse (or detach) from their thoughts and become less attached to their conceptualized or idealized self (Hayes, Luoma, Bond, Masuda, & Lillis, 2006). We use yoga in MYACT as an active form of mindfulness practice, and often, we use the breath as a metric for our connection to the present moment. As humans, we tend to push our body past its functional limits when we are mindless, and the breath—holding the breath or strained breath—cues us to this state.

There are a lot of ideas about what mindfulness is that may be contrary to or different from the way we approach our work. For example, many people conflate Buddhism and mindfulness. This is understandable, but there is an important distinction between Buddhist mindfulness and mindfulness as we know and practice it. Our version is informed by Patañjali's teachings and Tantrik philosophy.

On the one hand, mindfulness informed by Buddhist wisdom teaches the concept that there is no self, that all things are one, and therefore one cannot notice or create space between the self and individual experience because it is all one. The philosophies informing the yoga presented in MYACT, on the other hand, teach practitioners that there is a separation between the self and the content of one's experiences. From this perspective, we are able to be the observer of our thoughts, feelings, memories, and physical sensations (what in ACT we refer to as self-as-context), to make space for our thoughts and be open to all of our experiences (what in ACT we refer to as acceptance), and to gain distance from our thoughts by recognizing that thoughts are not rules or the capital T truth but simply content of the mind (what in ACT we refer to as defusion). Therefore, mindfulness in the context of MYACT can encompass a variety of different techniques, methods, or skills with a focus on training the six core processes of ACT's model, thus increasing psychological flexibility. At the core of the mindfulness we employ is the process of noticing.

As you begin to practice and train others in the practice of mindfulness, of noticing, it will be helpful to understand this distinction, as questions may arise during the eight-week protocol, or as you work with individual clients. Our aim in mindfulness is not to reach enlightenment, as is the goal in Buddhism, but rather to cultivate the practice of noticing our experience in this world. Being the observer of our experience can help us influence our behavior in the service of leading a meaningful life.

One simple way we cultivate this practice of noticing is through the breath. In yoga, the breath connects the mind, body, and environment. The events that happen throughout our day are being taken in by our senses and interpreted by our minds with thoughts, feelings, judgments, and reactions. The breath is constantly communicating with us about what we're experiencing, sometimes even before we're aware of it. For example, when people are anxious, they may hold their breath or breathe erratically.

In yogic philosophy, *prāṇāyāma* was classically described as the practice of controlling the breath. Although we begin to manipulate the movements of breathing—its timing, depth, and placement—in congruence with the model of psychological flexibility, we prefer the interpretation that prāṇāyāma is not the practice of controlling the breath but rather the practice of freeing the breath to move more fluidly and responsively within the body. To us, the goal of prāṇāyāma is to let the body breathe itself, to let the body breathe naturally. In fact, recent research has shown that deep-breathing practices, which are attempts to control breathing, can increase carbon dioxide levels in the body, creating sensations of dizziness or light-headedness. We do not encourage people to take deep breaths or to breathe in any particular way; rather, our instructions always focus on noticing the breath, connecting with the way it moves throughout the body, and allowing our breath to breathe naturally.

Prāṇāyāma can be a difficult practice for many, because as we practice watching the breath, sometimes we inadvertently attempt to manipulate it. That is why it is important for individuals to monitor how they feel while focusing on the breath, and it's important for instructors to provide instructions that reinforce uncontrolled breathing—that is, following the natural rhythm of the breath. If you or a participant starts to feel light-headed or dizzy, stop and relax and fall back to uncontrolled or effortless inhalations and exhalations (unless the purpose of the activity is to induce anxiety and panic symptoms as part of an exposure exercise in which sufficient informed consent has been given).

In MYACT and many other yogic traditions, we use the breath to focus present-moment attention on the body. The breath becomes a barometer for levels of stress and fatigue. The breath can show us when we're calm and when we're distracted. The beauty of breath in yoga is that it is a felt experience—one that can gently move our attention from other private experiences, beginning the work of focusing on other stimuli. You can't think breathing. You can think *about* breathing, generating judgments about your breath being shallow or deep, fast or slow. You can remember what the last breath you took felt like or fantasize what you want the next breath to feel like, but you can only experience the breath through the sensation of breathing in the body. The breath is a perfect introduction to the practice of noticing. Though many may struggle to identify thoughts or feelings, everyone can feel their breath expand and contract, even if that felt experience occurs in different places for different people.

Now that you have an understanding of the function of both mindfulness and the breath, as well as the necessary background information to explain them to others, let's look at the skeletal system, with an open mind and an eye for function. If this is a new area for you, take this section slowly. We included interactive exercises to both engage and demonstrate the importance of anatomy in our work.

Anatomy and Functional Movement

To perform or teach many of the yoga practices in this book requires an understanding of human anatomy: the basic structure of the body, posture, how the body's structure influences and limits alignment and positioning, and how the body moves. It's important to understand how a body moves and is meant to move relative to its structure. We present this section for purposes of utility, so you will know how to set up postures, how they work, and how to offer adjustments and modifications based on each individual body you work with. The goal is to keep the yoga practitioners in your program practicing safely. We use colloquial terms to refer to anatomical structures because the average person is not aware of the technical names for different parts of the body. As most psychotherapists don't spew jargon at their clients for obvious reasons, we believe that teachers and therapists are more effective when they avoid anatomical language in their instruction. Ultimately, our role is to offer you the tools necessary to effectively and safely practice and teach yoga while leaving out the components that aren't practical or necessary.

Basic Structure of the Body—the Skeleton

Understanding the underlying structure of the body can increase our ability to feel movement happening within our own body and to direct others in moving their own. In the sections that follow, we'll explore the skeletal system, from head to toe.

SKULL

In teaching yoga, the skull serves as a reference point for moving the neck and aligning the head. Colloquially we refer to the "crown of the head," meaning the top of the skull, when giving instructions, such as lengthening the spine. For example, right now as you're reading this book, reach through the crown of your head, lengthening through the neck, as if you had a string on the top of your head pulling you up. Notice the effect this has on your posture. During many postures, you will draw clients' attention to the alignment of their spine through the crown of their head to ensure proper form.

COLLARBONE (CLAVICLE)

The collarbones are a reference point when drawing the shoulder blades together by engaging the upper back. For example, draw your shoulder blades in toward your spine. Feel how the collarbones broaden as the upper back engages, creating more space. Notice sensations in the chest. Perhaps it feels broad or more open. Opening up our chest allows for deeper breath, slowing down, sinking into our poses, and attending to the positioning of our body.

SHOULDER BLADES (SCAPULAE)

Yoga instructions that involve the shoulder blades are often focused on how the body is aligned. When the shoulder blades are in good alignment, the arms will find a safe and efficient position. Finding a good shoulder position allows for a more sustainable posture. The yoga practitioner will not have to work as hard or be as physically challenged to maintain the pose.

For example, pause for a moment and raise your arms above your head, palms facing each other. The shoulder blades will naturally lift and rotate outwardly. Attempt to draw your shoulder blades away from your ears (this is a common cue in yoga classes when the arms are raised above the head, palms facing each other), and notice the sensations in your arms. Perhaps you notice a straining around the upper shoulders, the base of the neck, and the area around the bottom of your shoulder blades. Now, drop your arms, take a breath, and raise your arms again, but this time do so without attempting to pull your shoulder blades down. Notice the upward and outward movement of your shoulder blades as you lift the arms. This second position (upward and outward movement) tends to be a natural resting posture for modern-day people, who spend a lot of time hunched over computer screens, but it is anything but natural.

You'll find that drawing the shoulder blades away from the ears can be one of the most effective cues for adjusting postures. It's something that clients who are only able to practice seated yoga due to various physical disabilities can focus on to improve functional movement.

UPPER ARM BONE (HUMERUS)

The upper arm bone encompasses the area from the shoulder to the elbow. Because the arms frequently bear weight in yoga postures, their appropriate alignment is important. In postures that don't require the arms to bear weight, an awareness of the upper arm bones influences the stability and strength of the shoulders, contributing to a sustainable practice.

For example, take your arms out to the sides, forming a T position, with palms facing down. Internally rotate your arm bones so that the palms face backward and your thumbs point down. Notice sensations of cramping in the shoulders and upper neck. Now externally rotate your arm bones so that the palms face up and the thumbs face backward. Notice how the shoulder blades soften away from the ears and create a more sustainable strength in the shoulders. These small rotations can have a big impact, not only on strength and stability but on a person's belief in their ability to hold these postures.

When people say they've tried yoga and can't do it, this conclusion often is the result of dysfunctional movement patterns and alignment, which lead to feelings of tension and instability. Or sometimes it's the result of a teacher demonstrating or modeling a variation of movement that is simply not yet available to the participant due to limited mobility. People with past shoulder injuries or neck and shoulder pain often struggle with mobility. Instructing clients on the proper movements and positioning can increase their willingness to engage with yoga and can reinforce the practice of listening to the body.

FOREARM (RADIUS AND ULNA)

The forearm spans from the elbow to the wrist. Forearms influence proper hand and upper arm bone alignment in various postures. For example, take your arms out to the sides, forming a T position, with the palms facing down. Externally rotate the upper arm bones so that the palms face up. Now keep the upper arm bones externally rotated but begin to rotate the forearms so the palms to face down. Notice that if you start to overrotate through the forearm so that the palms start to face backward, the upper arm bone is pulled out of external rotation. You may even notice your shoulders beginning to curve inward, disrupting proper posture. This combination of movements is used to cue proper arm alignment in postures such as Downward Dog and Warrior 2.

HANDS

We often give specific instructions for what to do with the hands. They may be simple, such as spreading the fingers or facing the palms or thumbs in a certain direction, or complex, such as interlacing the fingers or pressing the base knuckle of the index finger into the floor.

In many yoga poses, the hands bear weight, which requires stability. To experience this, place the palm of one of your hands on a flat surface with your fingers together. Then, lightly spread the fingers and root down (press) through the base knuckle of the index finger. Feel how the palm engages, creating a stable and engaged hand. That stabilization is the base structure of the hands in many yoga poses, such as Table Top, Downward Dog, and Handstand, creating greater stability and distributing weight.

RIB CAGE

In practicing and teaching yoga, the ribs are essential for feeling the breath and as a reference point for positioning the shoulder blades or for feeling the movement of the rib cage in relation to the upper arm bones. For example, sit in a relaxed but upright position. Begin to draw the shoulder blades together, in toward the spine. Now draw the shoulder blades away from the spine. Without holding the breath, repeat this movement of drawing the shoulder blades together and then spreading them apart. Take the full length of an inhale to draw the shoulder blades together and the full length of an exhale to move the shoulder blades away from the spine. Notice sensations of the shoulder blades sliding on the rib cage.

An awareness of the shoulder blades sliding across the rib cage is used throughout MYACT to encourage functional movement. In being instructed to not hold your breath, you may have noticed you were doing just that—holding your breath while focusing on the movement. This is a common issue that arises as participants transition between and hold poses. Breath, as we've mentioned, is an important component of the experience and practice of yoga. As you continue to sit in your relaxed but upright position, take a long, slow, deep breath. Notice air filling the lungs and pushing out against the rib cage. If you don't feel this pressure, gently place one hand on your chest and one on your belly. Focus on pushing your lower hand out with each inhale and then, continuing to inhale, breathe into your chest, lifting your chest into your hand. You should be able to feel the breath filling up your lungs and pushing out against the rib cage. Sometimes it may feel as if your sides or upper back are expanding with each inhale.

STERNUM

The sternum is colloquially referred to as the "breastbone," but in our experience, most participants are familiar with the term "sternum," as it's often used in CPR. Used as a reference point for feeling rotation in the spine, the sternum is also used to cue lifting and lengthening through the upper spine. For example, seat yourself in an upright but relaxed position. Bring your hands to what we call heart center, so that your palms are together in a prayerlike position and your thumbs rest against the sternum. Begin to slowly twist your body to the right by rotating through the spine, keeping the lower body still. As you rotate, notice how the sternum moves with your twist. Release from the twist with an awareness of the sternum coming back to center. Now at the center position, reach up through the crown of your head, lifting the sternum. Notice the change in how you hold your body. The spine is more actively engaged, and the muscles in the back contract, providing more support and length to assist with better posture. Within the tallness of this posture, notice the sensation of the sternum lifting and falling on the inhale and exhale, guiding your awareness to this breathing. This posture can help you become more attuned to the relationship between the lungs, ribs, and sternum.

SPINE

Spinal health is one of the common goals of modern postural yoga because the spine is the central axis for all of the movements we do, and it holds all of the nerves that travel down the spinal canal. Therefore, it is difficult to live an active and functional life without a healthy spine. In yoga, the spine's alignment is targeted by flexing, extending, and twisting. The spine is also used as a common reference point in different postures for how it can be activated, such as describing the spine as "long and neutral" in Warrior 2 or "lengthened" in Chair. Take a moment now to work with spinal alignment cues.

From a seated position with the feet flat on the floor, begin to fold the torso (or upper body) over the thighs, noticing sensations of the spine rounding (flexing) as you do so. Return to an upright, neutral position, noticing the sensations of the spine extending. Yoga often engages both flexion and extension with complementary postures to encourage flexible movement that mirrors real life.

PELVIS

"Pelvis" is actually a general term that we use in yoga to describe several parts of the body: the ilium, which are pelvic bones on either side of the body; the sacrum that sits between the pelvic bones; the tailbone that sits at the bottom of the sacrum; and the ischium, commonly referred to as the sit bones. All of these parts are used as a reference point for either feeling movement in relation to other bones or in relation to an external landmark, such as squaring your pelvis to the floor or turning your pelvis toward the long end of the mat.

Take a moment to briefly explore the pelvis. Sit in a comfortable, upright position. Take the fingers of each hand and find the two bones on either side of your pelvis at the front. These bones are the front of your ilium. Now follow these bones toward the back of the body. You should feel a bony ridge as you travel back. As the hands get close together at the back, you should feel the bone protruding, creating bumps. This is the back of the ilium. In between those two bumps is the top of your sacrum. Relax your arms. Now feel the bones you are sitting on, the sit bones. Shift from side to side so they become more apparent. You may wish to move the flesh aside (adjusting your butt cheeks) to experience your sit bones making contact with the surface you're sitting on.

Now, explore how the pelvis moves. Start by imagining your pelvis is like a bowl. Tilt your pelvis forward as though you want to spill water out of the front of the bowl. Notice how the weight shifts to the front of the sit bones. Now tilt the pelvis in the opposite direction as though you are spilling water out of the back of the bowl. Notice again how the weight shifts on the sit bones, this time toward the back. Moving the pelvis may also impact your balance and the position of your spine. Try that tilting pattern a few more times, spilling the water forward and then backward. Also, notice how the spine responds and shifts as you tilt the pelvis. We will use this movement and awareness of the pelvis tilting as a foundation for building more complex yoga postures in the MYACT protocol.

THIGH BONES (FEMURS)

The thigh bones, or femurs, are the largest bones in the human body—and for good reason. They support the weight of the entire pelvis and upper body. These bones are also important for locomotion, and they're critical for nearly every posture in yoga, especially standing balance postures.

Come to a standing position to briefly explore the kinds of movements the thigh bones can express. If balance is a safety concern for you, or you would prefer some support in this posture, consider leaning against a wall. Start by drawing your right thigh bone up toward the abdomen, allowing the right knee to bend. Return the foot to the floor. Now, move the right leg back behind you, keeping the leg straight as you do. Again, return the foot to the floor. Now, lift the right leg to the side. Return it to the floor. Repeat this movement pattern on the left side. Notice if you can feel which muscles are contracting to make these movements happen. In MYACT, the thigh bones and legs are important landmarks for many postures.

SHIN BONES (TIBIA AND FIBULA)

The shin bones comprise the area between the knee and the ankle. In yoga, the shins are commonly used as an anatomical landmark for positioning the knee joint in relation to the ankle. For example, in lunges, participants are instructed to stack the knee over the ankle so that the shin bones are in a vertical position. In Boat, participants are instructed to position the shin bones parallel to the floor, so they serve as a landmark in relation to the floor.

Take a moment to explore the shin bones. Find an upright seated position with your feet flat on the floor. Close your eyes. Without looking at your feet or shins, try to determine whether or not your ankles are directly underneath your knees, so that your shin bones are perpendicular to the floor, or if the ankles are a little bit forward of the knees or behind them. Once you have a pretty good guess in your mind, open your eyes and look at your shins. How accurate were you? If the shins are perpendicular, great, your proprioception (the awareness of the position or movement of your body in relation to your surroundings) is likely very strong. If not, adjust the feet so the shins are straight up and down, close your eyes, and take a moment to notice what that experience is like in the body. Notice the position of your knees in relation to the shins, and the shins in relation to the ankles and feet.

FEET

Our feet hold us up and propel us forward and backward, and as such, their placement and use is important in yoga. The primary function of the feet, anatomically, is stability, and yet feet also need to remain flexible and mobile. Feet are durable and yet need to remain sensitive so they can more easily pick up information from the ground. One of the primary benefits of yoga is that it's typically done with bare feet. This allows them to pick up more data pertaining to the surface they are in contact with. In turn, they send signals to the brain, which then cues other areas of the body, such as the core or the hips, to align themselves with the rest of the body.

Come to a standing position with bare feet. If balance is a concern or you would like additional support, place one hand on a stable surface, such as a table, chair, or wall. Lift one foot off the floor. Notice how the opposite foot, ankle, leg, and hip, and the core, automatically have to do more work. Keep the breath soft and smooth. Draw your attention to the sole of your standing foot. Feel for what we call the three corners of the foot: ball of the big toe, ball of the baby toe, and the center of the heel. Notice how the pressure from the body's weight fluctuates at these three corners. Also notice how when you start to move out of balance, one of these three corners lifts or the ankle moves in or out as weight shifts. When you begin to fall off-balance, be curious about how your body attempts to compensate, perhaps by tightening the upper body, holding the breath, or using the arms to correct the imbalance. Using the arms for assistance is not a bad thing. However, instead of using the arms to correct your balance, try making the adjustment at the foot and ankle. The ability to bring more awareness to the feet can assist your balance on and off the yoga mat.

JOINTS

Joints are the places in the body where bones meet. For example, the knee joint is where the femur of the upper leg meets the tibia and fibula of the lower leg. A facet joint in the spine is where one vertebra meets another.

Healthy joint function is one of the underlying goals of modern postural yoga. A healthy joint is one that can express a good degree of movement, relative to its location, and can function while being supported by the surrounding musculature. Contrary to popular belief, yoga is not solely about getting flexible or putting your foot behind your head. Yoga is about creating a balance between flexibility, strength, and stability. This is why in MYACT, we don't stress pushing too hard in a pose or movement. When yoga practices go wrong, practitioners often overextend their joints or twist in ways that strain natural movement by going beyond the purpose of the pose. In MYACT, we are not focused on hitting that "perfect" pose.

Functional Movements and Cues

In MYACT, the main focus with movement is not whether the yoga pose looks like the instructor's or some cool photo, but rather if movement is expressed within the mobility available to the participant. This is the definition of functional movement. Now that you have a working knowledge of the different parts of the body, we'll demonstrate how those parts are meant to move, as well as their range of available movement. We have included common cues, or language, used in yoga practice to help participants notice how their body is moving and to appropriately make adjustments based on function and mobility.

Biomechanics and Planes of Movement

The laws of biomechanics are relatively simple. Every joint is a meeting place where two or more bones come together. Depending on the shape of the bones coming together, each joint is designed to move in specific ways. For example, the knee joint has only two movements (flexion and extension) available and is known as a hinge joint. The shoulder joint, however, has six available movements and is known as a ball-and-socket joint. It allows an arm to move in many ways.

The body can be divided by imaginary lines called anatomical planes, and joints move in relation to these lines in what's called planular movement. There are three anatomical planes: sagittal, frontal, and transverse. The sagittal plane divides the body into right and left, the frontal plane into front and back, and the transverse plane into upper and lower. The benefit of knowing and understanding the basic principles of biomechanics and planular movement is that you can then teach people how to move better and reduce the risk of injury.

Movements and Their Planes

Flexion is movement in a joint that results in the angle between two bones getting smaller. The opposing movement is known as *extension*, in which the angle of the joint gets larger. Both of these are sagittal plane movements. Flexion and extension are available in every major joint of the body. Looking at the simple act of kicking a soccer ball might help make this more clear. Extension happens when we draw the leg back (the angle between the front of the pelvis and the thigh bone gets larger), and flexion occurs when we bring the leg forward to kick the ball (the angle between the pelvis and thigh becomes shorter).

Abduction is the sideways movement of a limb away from the midline of the body—for instance, when you move your arms out and away from your body. Conversely, *adduction* is the movement of a limb toward the midline of the body—for instance, when you bring your outstretched arms back to your sides. Both of these are frontal plane movements, which are available primarily in the shoulders and hips.

Internal and *external rotation* are movements involving the upper arm bone or thigh bone rotating inwardly or outwardly in its socket. This movement happens through the transverse plane. To explore internal rotation in the upper arm, start with your arms resting at your sides. Imagine that there is a dot in the middle of each of your biceps. Then, rotate the upper arms so that the dots point inward toward the midline. Relax the arms back to center. Try this movement a few more times to become more familiar with how it feels in your body.

Posture

Historically, if people stood tall with good posture, it meant something profound about them. That they carried themselves in this way suggested status, confidence, or strength and was a reflection of their personal qualities. In gyms and yoga studios the world over you'll still hear people talking about how form is important, and it's true. It's also essential to know that "good" form doesn't necessarily equal good function, as it was once thought to. Good form or good posture is a product of the underlying function of the body. If the function of the body is poor, the posture will be poor by consequence. If the function is good, the posture will reflect that.

Within MYACT, we focus more on the function of the body, using movement and breathing as the primary barometers for how we approach any given movement or posture. Why? Because, again, forcing the body into "good" form without regard for the underlying functional abilities of the body or structure can lead to injury. This approach and focus on function will allow you to work more intimately with your clients because you'll be working with how their body functions rather than trying to make their body adhere to a posture or a specific set of alignments, just hoping that things work out. It also creates a sense of acceptance around whatever the body is capable of doing in the moment and encourages clients to practice listening to their own body, both within the practice of yoga and outside in their everyday movements and life.

Common Cues and What They Mean

Below, we've listed common cues we use within the practice of asana (and in this book) that might seem vague. Although they refer to a direction of movement and a body part, the terms we use are not technically anatomical ones.

- "Reach through the crown of the head" refers to the top of the head (crown) lifting or moving away from the base of the spine in order to lengthen the back and to help decrease excessive rounding in the upper spine. If participants are standing, we might follow this cue with imagery of someone lightly pulling on a string attached to the top of the skull.

- "Long neutral spine" refers to the natural curves of the spine. Depending on the posture, a client may have the tendency to slouch and excessively round (flex) the spine or, at the opposite end of the spectrum, have too much extension in either the neck or low back. This cue to lengthen from these positions of excess can help bring the spine back to a more neutral place, potentially creating the conditions for other parts of the body (including the diaphragm) to move more efficiently.

- "Fold" and "hinge" refer specifically to moving the pelvis in relation to the thigh bones. For instance, in Standing Full-Sun Salutation we might cue to "Inhale, reach the arms up. Exhale to *fold* forward over the top of the thighs," or "Exhale to *hinge* at the hip and fold the body forward."

- "Root down" describes a body part or series of parts pushing into the surface that clients are in contact with. For example, "*Root* the feet down into the floor" is a common instruction for participants in a standing posture, and "Root down evenly from the shoulders and armpits into the palms of the hands" for postures such as Table or Downward Dog.

- "Craning the neck" refers to an overextended position of the cervical spine. In class we might say something like "Inhale, raise the arms up, taking the gaze toward the hands but without *craning the neck* or trying to look up to the point of discomfort."

Preparing to Teach MYACT

In this chapter, we demonstrated how teaching yoga involves integrating knowledge of anatomy, skeletal and muscular structure, and planes of movement. We provided cues for helping participants to see their movements from a functional perspective and to make appropriate adjustments based on their body. In MYACT, we don't offer any one alignment for the "correct" asana. Instead, we prompt functional movement with these cues, which encourage variation and a scaling of difficulty for the postures. As you move through the MYACT protocol, we encourage you to apply our cues to your own personal practice. Notice how your body responds to them so you're better prepared to teach MYACT to others.

Congratulations! You have all of the theoretical, philosophical, and anatomical information necessary to begin learning and implementing the MYACT eight-week protocol. Part 2 will walk you through how to bring MYACT to life.

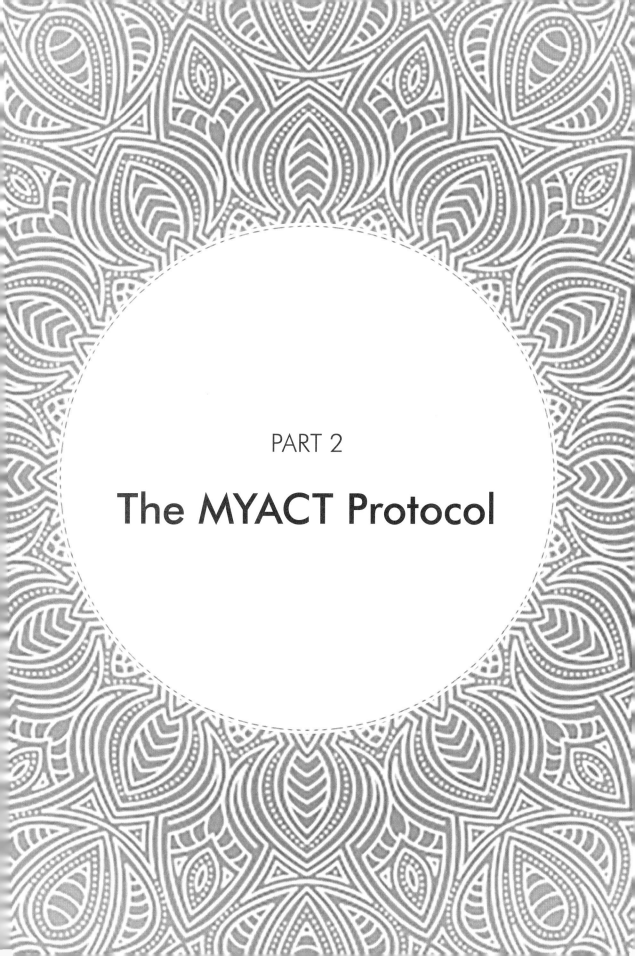

PART 2

The MYACT Protocol

In part 2, we're going to focus on the process of doing mindful yoga-based ACT in direct practice, leaving the theoretical, philosophical, and conceptual issues behind. Please feel free to return to the chapters in part 1 to clarify process-based issues. In the following pages, we offer reasons for focusing on specific concepts in each session, as well as suggestions for how to become flexible yourself in how you present MYACT.

Before moving forward with this book, we offer this recommendation: read all eight sessions before you use MYACT for the first time so you have a sense of how the protocol is structured. The concepts of each session build and flow into the next session, building a larger whole. The idea is to approach every moment from a place of flexibility.

While we may emphasize a particular psychological flexibility skill in each session, we don't want to imply that you should only use this one skill in the session, such as acceptance for session one, defusion for session two, and so forth. Depending on context, use whichever skill seems most appropriate for the moment. For example, if someone is talking fast or interrupting, slow down very purposefully to help them come in contact with the present moment, and try to notice what is driving their behavior (for example, maybe they're uncomfortable with the topic of values because they feel disconnected from theirs, so they begin to rush through the conversation or talk in tangents as a way to avoid discomfort). You may want to exaggerate certain poses to highlight and draw attention to the process of noticing, or a faster pace may be appropriate to help clients engage with a posture and feel different physical sensations. This process requires some flexibility on your part rather than rigid adherence to the protocol.

There are scripts throughout the protocol; however, you may want to modify them to fit examples clients have mentioned, or you may want to break from the scripts. For example, if a client reports struggling with focusing on physical sensations in a meditation, spend additional time doing so rather than blindly moving forward with the script. Let the context dictate the work. We do recommend that you read all of the scripts out loud, practice them with your own inflection, and make them your own so you can use them with fluidity.

Group Composition

MYACT is a flexible intervention, suitable for one-on-one work and work in groups alike. In this book, we have written and structured the protocol for use in groups, with guidance on adaptations for individuals given at the end of each session. While we understand that some of you may work primarily with individuals, we encourage you, if possible, to consider the benefits and possibilities of running groups. One major benefit of group work for clients is the realization that they aren't alone. In isolation, it's easy to assume that you are the only one struggling with a problem and therefore there is something wrong with you or you are weird or broken in some way. Even in groups with mixed presenting problems (for example, anxiety, chronic pain, depression, health concerns), the sharing, support, and recognition of universal patterns of responding encourages clients to open up more to the process. Through the group process they also gain a level of confidence in their ability to learn and implement new strategies in their lives, rather than simply admitting defeat. It's a beautiful process to watch unfold. Additionally, compared to individual work, groups generally have a lower cost per session, and offering group sessions may help you reach those who are unable to afford private sessions or who might be dismissive of individual therapy but open to a group environment.

As you can tell, we're big fans of group work! If you're not, don't worry, everything in the MYACT protocol can be modified to fit individual needs and varying settings or session lengths. Regardless of how you run the MYACT protocol, there is some general information you should know before diving in.

You may experience a large amount of variability in who attends MYACT individual or group sessions, and that's fine. You don't need to conduct separate MYACT sessions for social anxiety and shyness and chronic pain. We have found strong cohesion in groups with varying presenting concerns, ages, sexualities and gender identities, and levels of ability. And since we are looking at how behaviors function rather than simply at symptoms presented, you'll find that the patterns of avoidance for different clients are similar, even if the manifestation of that avoidance looks different from the outside.

Variability in composition can also encourage generative learning. Clients may begin to see how processes, perspectives, and approaches to their issues can be applied to other problems they may face in the future, or to better understand the actions of people in their lives. This is a powerful ability, as it means the impact of this protocol will last after the sessions end and the approach and new way of interacting with their world can spread beyond just the clients that make up your group.

Settings and Props

The MYACT protocol is flexible. It can be done in a traditional therapy room as part of individual therapy or at a yoga studio, a recreational room at a hospital or gym, or a group therapy space. For the group protocol, all you need is a space that accommodates each participant and their standard yoga mat, and maybe some wiggle room so folks have the chance to move around if needed. Here are some other items that we recommend:

- **Dry-erase board:** We use this for some of our exercises, such as doing a group life map. A large flip board with markers, a chalkboard, or one of those fancy electronic whiteboards with a large-presentation setup works as well.

- **Yoga mat:** Generally, we have participants buy their own. We emphasize that there is no need for expensive high-end yoga mats that cost $100. Rather, they can pick one up for a couple of dollars that works just fine. We have even done yoga on large towels in a conference room or on a carpeted floor, though yoga mats can allow for a more structured (and comfortable) setting.

- **Pillows or folded-up towels or blankets:** These can provide relief for clients with a limited range of mobility or pain in certain parts of the body. For example, we may suggest that clients with back pain put a folded towel under the knees when they are lying on their back in Savasana. For seated practices, some sit on a pillow or folded towel or blanket to slightly raise their hips and ease any pain a cross-legged position may entail.

- **Yoga blocks:** Clients can use these foam bricks to assist with balance. For example, in Side Angle pose, they may put the block on the floor and prop themselves up with it to maintain a functional posture rather than straining or losing form for the sake of touching the ground.

- **Straps:** Clients who struggle with range of motion issues may find these valuable. The strap can act as a bridge between a person's hand and whatever other body part they are trying to touch, such as if they are trying to clasp their hands behind their back but their hands can't reach. Remember, though, there is no need to spend a lot of money; chairs and walls work for balance, too.

Collaboration

Yoga teachers will likely find themselves out of their comfort zone and scope of practice while running the eight-week MYACT protocol. Similarly, mental health professionals may be hesitant to instruct yoga poses on their own. Though Tim is both a registered social worker and a trained yoga instructor, when he first began running the eight-week MYACT protocol, he approached yoga instructors, like Steve, to help him run the protocol. Tim and Steve together have regularly run the protocol, allowing both of their unique strengths to be reflected in one transformative group. As Steve has become more comfortable with the ACT language, he has taken a larger role in the discussion-centered parts of sessions, and Tim often leads yoga practices, but it was a process for them to reach this point.

While it is in no way mandatory, we encourage yoga teachers and mental health professionals to team up and collaborate through the MYACT protocol. Doing so provides wonderful opportunities to connect with and learn from peers. Yoga studios and mental health clinics and hospitals often have access to and knowledge of different resources available to clients. When you pool your resources and knowledge, you become like the protocol: greater than the sum of its parts. In order to facilitate such collaborations, we have developed a MYACT Facebook group for people who have read this book or completed our online course or our yoga teacher training. Through it, you can connect, ask questions, and share experiences with others. If after reading this book you would like to connect online with us, go to http://www.facebook.com/groups/MYACT. Also, if you have concerns regarding the scope of practice, chapter 6 is dedicated to this topic.

Logically, we find ourselves giving you one last piece of professional practice advice. This second part of MYACT, its session protocol, is a skeleton. We don't debate that if you attempt to follow it verbatim you're likely to get good results, but the organic nature of this work will have been lost on you. MYACT is a living, breathing practice that we intend for you to model as a MYACT facilitator. If you substitute exercises, deconstruct scripts, and model appropriate use of self by revealing your feelings of hope, loss, regret, sadness, and merriment in MYACT, you'll likely have succeeded in doing something important and arguably essential: lived this work yourself. Learn from the protocol, yes, but don't be afraid to make it your own.

Each MYACT session has a theme based on a yogic concept. These concepts bridge yoga practices with ACT processes and exercises to facilitate in-session experiential learning. They also prepare clients for generalizing what they're learning in the MYACT group to their out-of-session life.

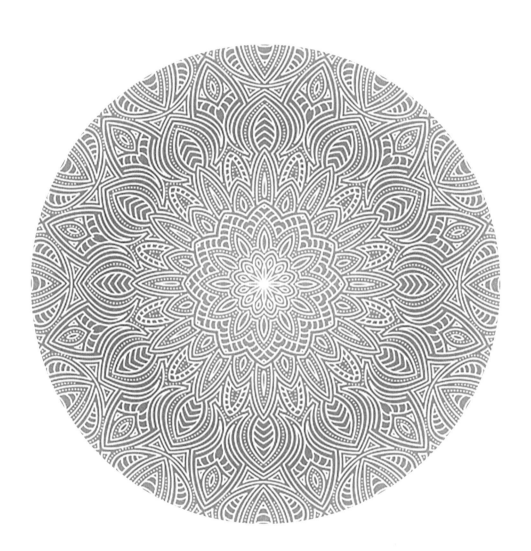

Dhāranā

The first session of MYACT is thematically based on the yogic concept of *dhāranā*, meaning "focus" or "one-pointed attention." With dhāranā, participants are shown multiple examples of how to focus their awareness by moving from distraction to attention. We encourage them to use this newfound process to recognize conditioned patterns of distraction, as noticing is the first step in changing how we interact with the world and ourselves. The mind arising from different directions and leading to distraction or attachment to experiences and outcomes, or *vyutthāna samskāra*, is an important concept in yoga. This ability to get lost in our mind, or to become fixated on a certain outcome (such as happiness), is an evolutionary feature of our species. It enhanced our ability to survive by allowing us to detect threats, as within our minds we can imagine future scenarios, identify potential barriers or threats to survival, and determine how to overcome them to reach a desired outcome. While this ability can be helpful at times, it also takes us away from our lived experience. Yoga's prescription of dhāranā is a simple answer to this problem: learn to be fully present, focusing attention on the now.

We begin the introduction to dhāranā with practices for creating a shared space of safety, mutuality, and equal vulnerability. Throughout the MYACT protocol you will notice a liberal use of self-disclosure on the facilitators' part. This is purposeful. Facilitators model psychological flexibility in the way they conduct themselves in the group and functionally self-disclose their own struggles. Obviously, this is done to the extent you feel comfortable, and with a functional purpose.

Begin this first session by welcoming participants, giving a brief introduction to the space the group will be practicing in (explain where to find water, changing areas, bathrooms, emergency exits), and explaining practical details, such as where yoga mats should be placed and that this first group begins with them simply sitting on their mats and waiting for the group to commence.

Orientation

The facilitator or someone else (a receptionist or designated individual) welcomes the participants, invites them to enter the room where the yoga group will be conducted, and asks them to remove shoes and socks and sit on a yoga mat. The participants' mats should be set up in a circle, with the facilitator's mat included as a part of the group, generally close to the front of the room. (Alternatively, if the space is too small to accommodate a circle, the mats can be set up in rows during yoga. Participants can then be invited to get up off their mats and sit in a circle for group discussions.) Ideally, the group will have no more than twelve participants. In our experience, it's easiest to have mats already placed on the floor in the orientation that you wish before participants arrive. Participants who bring their own mat can layer their own over another or replace a mat with their own. Instruct them that this is how the group will be set up for every meeting.

Welcome participants and ask them to find a comfortable way to sit. Briefly outline the first session: "We'll begin with introductions, do a group exercise, practice yoga, and do another exercise before we finish for the day." Explain confidentiality, including its limits, and explain how participants should choose their own level of participation. We've had a lot of success emailing informed consent and confidentiality forms in advance and having participants sign and turn them in before they enter the session space.

Describe yoga as a nonreligious practice. "Yoga is free from deities or any requirement of worship. This is a nonreligious practice that can be used by people who wish to use yoga as a way of expressing their spirituality, but this is not how we will direct you to practice yoga in MYACT."

This is a good time to let participants know what ACT is (said aloud as "act"), that it stands for acceptance and commitment therapy (or "training," if the facilitator is not a mental health professional; see chapter 6 for a discussion on scope of practice). In ACT, the mantra is that actions change things. Let participants know that ACT is a way of learning about how our minds work, and that it encourages us to look at the struggles our minds can create in our life. Make clear that ACT is about how we can live life in a way that is true to what we value most without struggling against the mind, but instead working with it.

You may wish to use this sample welcome script for MYACT at the opening of your first session:

> Welcome to MYACT. In this first session, we're going to introduce ourselves to one another and talk about what we want this group to be about. MYACT is based on acceptance and commitment therapy [or training], abbreviated as ACT and said aloud as the word "act." What we mean by "acceptance" is learning how to struggle less with the things that have long caused us to suffer, and to learn how to make commitments to the things that will help us connect in new ways to the life we most want for ourselves.

Our philosophy in this protocol is that what we do, the ways that we behave and interact with the world, is important, and that our actions change things. Throughout this group, we're going to ask you to participate in a number of different ways, including talking to one another in a group, physically doing the practice of yoga, and completing a number of different personal exercises. We'd like to encourage your participation but know that some of what we will ask of you may be outside your comfort zone. Choose your own level of participation. Know that a totally valid way of participating in this work may be to sit back and just observe the group process.

Before moving on to the introduction exercise, we recommend explaining the experiential nature of the group and describing group norms and expectations about how participants will behave in the group. For example, we tell participants that this is an experiential group that involves sharing difficult experiences and doing practices that will likely evoke difficult thoughts, feelings, sensations, or memories. We often joke that our only expectation is that participants aren't offensive toward the group, including the facilitator. If they choose to only observe a practice, we ask that they don't get in the way of the group process. Furthermore, before conducting group exercises, we're careful to explain what will happen during the exercise and what each participant will be asked to do. Our hope is that by giving participants adequate information, their decision to participate is considered informed consent.

Introduction and Intention-Setting Exercise

Ask group members to briefly introduce themselves, one by one: "Introduce yourself with your name and what your experience level is with yoga, including none at all if you've never done yoga. And then share what you most hope to get from this group."

You might begin by introducing yourself, your history with yoga, and what you hope to get from the group before asking the participant seated closest to you to do the same, then moving along one by one in sequence through all of the participants. Alternatively, we've had success running groups with two facilitators. One of the facilitators begins, followed by each of the participants, before ending with the other facilitator sharing.

We use a whiteboard to collect answers. We write down participants' names and their hoped outcomes, or intentions, from the group. We take a picture of the whiteboard because we'll return to this intention setting later in this first session, with the group life map, and during the final session. Alternatively, you may wish to have participants write their names and hopes for the group on a piece of paper as a letter to themselves and then place their responses in an envelope to be opened in the final session.

Thanking the group for their participation, transition from the group discussion, seated on yoga mats, to the first yoga practice, a resting posture called Savasana. "We're going to do a brief yoga practice with a simple posture. At the beginning of every group, when you return to this space, set yourselves up on your mat in silence in this pose. That is how we'll start every session from now on."

Beginning with Savasana: Bringing Your Whole Self to the Room

Instruct participants to lay down flat on their back, arms at their sides, palms facing up, and feet splayed out.

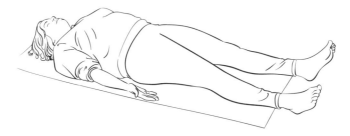

For those who may be suffering with low back pain, we suggest they slightly bend the knees and place blocks or a blanket beneath them for support, or have them plant their feet flat on the mat with a block between their legs and a strap wrapped around them.

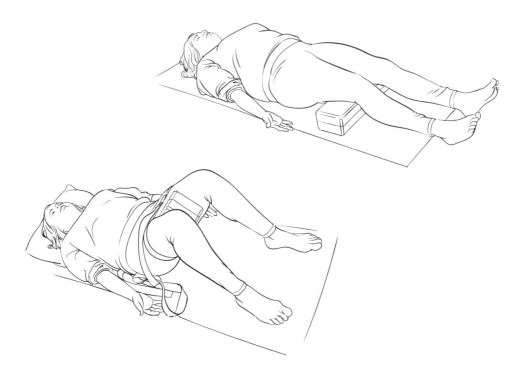

During this first yoga posture of MYACT, we don't offer to physically adjust participants, and we allow them time to settle into the practice. Here's a script we use for this first meditation on bringing one's whole self to the room.

As you settle into this first posture, take a breath on purpose and notice the sensations of breath in your body.

Notice how the belly expands as you inhale and collapses on the exhale.

Inevitably distractions show up, whether there are sounds or sensations you notice in your body. On your next inhale, scan your experience and notice those distractions. Exhale to bring your focus right back to the sensations of breath in the body. Inhale to notice thoughts and feelings, maybe even thoughts about the fact that you're distracted. Perhaps you're saying to yourself, *I'm not supposed to be thinking about this!* Whatever shows up, inhale to breathe it in and exhale to come back to the sensations of breath, noticing where you feel your breath in your body.

And just breathe.

On your next inhale, notice how, as the body fills with air, it just seems to know when it's had enough air. There's a natural point where air stops moving into the body. You don't even need to think about it. See if, as you inhale, you can catch that natural pause.

On the next inhale, as your body fills with air and pauses, see if you can take an extra breath in, topping off the lungs with oxygen before exhaling all the way.

And notice what that feels like in the body.

Repeat this pausing, focusing your attention on the body's natural pause and taking an extra breath. If you find yourself becoming distracted, bring your attention right back to this movement of breath and your ability to draw in extra air at your natural pause.

As you're present here with your breath, invite your whole self to come to this room and join the rest of the people here in this group, who are also bringing their whole selves to the group. And breathe here, just noticing what your mind might tell you.

Bringing your whole self to this experience means bringing your hopes for yourself and your doubts, your cynicism, and your heart, allowing your vulnerabilities and your kindness to be present here.

And before we end this exercise, just take a brief moment to notice what it feels like to be in this moment, to have your whole self invited to this room. And if your mind tries to tell you *Yeah, that's great, but I could never say this or tell them that other thing*, just notice that, breathe, and come back to the present moment without a need to get caught up in distractions.

Still with your eyes closed, bring your attention back to the room we're in. Noticing sounds, noticing the sensations of the earth beneath you supporting your body.

Bring a little motion to the body, wiggling the fingers, rotating the wrists, wiggling the toes, rotating the ankles. Maybe turning the head from side to side. When you feel ready, allow the eyes to flutter open, rolling to the right side and using your left hand to prop yourself up so that you may come back to being seated on your mat, rejoining the group.

Seat yourself at the front of your yoga mat, in silence, waiting for each participant to return to a seated posture and rejoin the group. Look from one participant to the next, perhaps making eye contact with each to visually check in. We then commonly ask, "What did you notice?" Give participants time to share their experience. Sometimes more prompting is required, and we may ask, "As you were doing that exercise, what thoughts, feelings, sensations, memories, or distractions showed up for you? There's no wrong answer."

That last comment about there not being a wrong answer is true. That said, oftentimes participants tell us the exercise felt *good* or tell us it was *relaxing*. Keep in mind that this is not the aim of the activity. Still, whether a participant tells you an exercise felt good or shares that a sound or thought was distracting and made it difficult to focus, thank them for sharing their experience, whatever that experience happened to be. Ultimately, the aim is to pay attention, noticing all of our experiences—pleasant, unpleasant, or otherwise—and participants who offer such answers have done so. Debriefing this first Savasana practice is a helpful way to socialize participants to the work of noticing, which we'll also be doing with the life map.

Group Life Map

We had you, the reader, complete your very own life map in part 1 of this book, and now it's time to facilitate it with others. This is a quick and easy, hands-on way of delivering all six processes of ACT while training participants in how to recognize their own unworkable patterns of avoidance. You might introduce the exercise this way:

When describing what this protocol is about, I told you that what we do matters, and this exercise is about creating a map of our lives, both the private experiences you have, such as thoughts, feelings, memories, and physical sensations, as well as the ways you interact with the world and people around you. We put you at the center of the life map because it's about you, the experiences you notice and the things you do.

We typically use a whiteboard, flip chart, or a wireless device connected to a projector to facilitate the life map with a group. We draw a horizontal line with arrowheads on each side and begin with quadrant 1, values, in the bottom right.

Quadrant 1: Values. Pose this question to the group: "Who is most important to you? No need to be polite, just shout out your answers and I'll try to keep up." We write their answers in the bottom-right quadrant. If participants are sheepish when answering, we'll share our answers out loud and write them down. If you have two facilitators, it can be helpful for the person not at the board to shout out their answers to encourage others to share. When a group is hesitant to respond or one or two people take over the conversation, we may work our way through the group asking each participant to name one to two people who matter to them.

We then ask, "Apart from who is important to you, what is important to you? What qualities do you want to be about?" At this point, we tend to get fairly rich answers. One person might say work is important, whereas another might say faith or nature. We have had a lot of success pointing at the name of a child or parent that someone listed earlier and asking, "What kind of parent or partner do you want to be?" We finish by polling the group: "By a show of hands, does everyone see at least one example of who and what are important to you?" If someone doesn't raise their hand, inquire what you can add to the list that would resonate with them. We believe that to connect with the exercise as a whole, every participant should see one example of who or what is important to them.

> **Pro Tip:** Some clients might respond with answers like "be happy" or "be at peace." Since our goal is not to create or reduce certain emotions—and we have no way of guaranteeing happiness all the time—we want to look out for these types of responses and dig a little deeper. You may write down "be happy" as a value, but follow up with a question: "And if you were living a happy life, what would that look like?" For example, a person may then respond with "take more camping trips with the family, and exercise more." You could then ask what's important about camping trips (nature, spending time with family, teaching children survival skills) and exercise (health, being able to do more things with their children, and so on). This line of inquiry not only helps you identify values for individual participants, but it helps the entire group learn how to begin to examine their own life to see what is important to them.

Quadrant 2: Painful private content. Once we have established a list—it doesn't have to be exhaustive—of who and what are most important to participants, we contrast this with the thoughts, feelings, sensations, and memories that make it hard to engage with these values. We do this by first pointing to the bottom-left quadrant and asking, "What shows up for you that makes it hard to engage with the people and qualities in your life that matter to you? We're talking about the painful thoughts, feelings, sensations, and memories that show up for you."

The variety of answers that arises in this context is nearly endless, though look out for answers based on external obstacles, such as "My professional mentor Ben was a despotic asshole." When these sorts of answers come up, we don't question the merits of the argument but instead direct the participant's attention to thoughts, feelings, sensations, and memories: "What makes dealing with your mentor hard for you personally? What experience—thoughts, feelings, physical sensations, memories—show up and make interacting with him especially painful?" While we recognize people can cause pain in our lives, we want to identify which private experience shows up in relation to that person. It might be anger or disappointment or a traumatic memory.

Pay attention to balance, too. Ideally, the group will come up with examples of all four categories of internal experience. If a group is offering a lot of feelings, for example, but not giving examples of thoughts or sensations or memories, you might ask questions that steer them to consider the categories they're neglecting. The goal here is to train participants to notice the entirety of their private experience. For example, some may find it easy to identify feelings but struggle to identify thoughts. You can point this out and ask, "When this feeling shows up do you notice if any physical sensations show up too?" or "When you have this feeling, imagine a big thought bubble above your head. What does that thought bubble say?" By doing so, you are helping that person learn new ways to identify different experiences that are related.

Quadrant 3: Avoidance strategies. We then transition to the top-left quadrant by asking the group, "When these painful experiences show up in your life, what do you do to attempt to escape, avoid, or control them?" Answers often include substance abuse, consuming media such as television or web series, avoiding people by not attending social situations or answering phone calls, having sex, eating, or sleeping. When someone provides a vague or abstract answer such as "I shut down," we write that down but follow up with "What does that look like? If I were hanging out with you, what would I see you do?" Coming to this group, going to therapy, doing yoga, and meditating are answers that could also go in this quadrant. We are explicit that not all the behaviors listed in this quadrant are strictly problematic. In fact, you may find that people are hesitant to honestly share their more unattractive behaviors, so this could be an opportunity for one of the facilitators to share their own responses.

> **Pro Tip:** Sometimes participants are thrown off by the phrase "attempt to escape, avoid, or control" because they don't know what it means. If participants are struggling to come up with responses for quadrant 3, you may prompt them by pointing to something written in the bottom-left quadrant. "I noticed a couple people nodded their heads when Rachel said she has the thought 'What's the

point? Nothing will ever change.' If I were—in a noncreepy way—watching you as this thought popped up, what would I see you do next?" This line of inquiry focuses participants to identify observable behaviors that occur in response to a specific private experience.

On the other hand, some people may tend toward cognitive avoidance strategies when painful content shows up, such as ruminating, thinking about "what if" scenarios, or analyzing a thought or memory. If a participant responds to the question with "You would see me sitting on my couch staring at the wall," you might follow up with "Okay, thanks for responding. When you're sitting on your couch staring at the wall, what is your mind doing?" They may respond with "thinking what would have happened if only I had done better at my last job," or "thinking through all the ways I'd have to be different in order for someone to want to date me." This gives you the opportunity to highlight what's happening in this moment: "I see, so when this painful thought shows up you tend to start generating 'what if' scenarios or analyzing your life. Can I write those down? They're kind of like mental behaviors you do to avoid or escape that painful thought. Your mind takes you somewhere else."

Quadrant 4: Committed actions. It's easy to transition to the top-right quadrant by asking, "If you weren't spending your time and energy attempting to avoid, escape, and control your pain, what could you be doing or are already doing that helps you chase a life that's important to you?" We find it especially helpful to orient participants' attention back to the individual values in the bottom-right quadrant, perhaps reading them aloud before soliciting answers about behaviors to list in the top-right quadrant: "If I could see you connecting with [value] more, what would that look like?" These behaviors do not have to be drastic or extreme. They can be small and simple, such as sending a text message to a friend, packing an apple with lunch, or asking a partner how their day was.

The next step is to ask what it feels like to try and avoid, escape, or control the painful experiences in life. You may get a variety of answers. Most people say it doesn't feel good or is stressful, but sometimes, people say doing so feels good or provides relief. This is normal. Remember, they wouldn't be doing these behaviors if they didn't work in at least some small way. Next, contrast noticing what it feels like to try to avoid, escape, or control with what it feels like to chase the life that's important to them. The answers we get range from peaceful, amazing, and good to scary, stressful, and bad. It's good to emphasize that engaging in behaviors that move us toward a life that's important can feel risky: "Living a life connected with values isn't always easy, and sometimes it feels downright terrifying."

Finish the life map by reiterating that participants are at the center of it. "When you're at the mall looking at the directory to find a certain store, there is always a little red dot or a gold star on the map. What does it say?" Typically, many participants jump in and say, "You are here!" We smile, write "You are here" in the center of the star at the middle of the life map, and say, "You are here, that's right. We put you at the middle of the life map because it's a map to who and what matter to you. It shows you behaviors that connect you with these values but also the hazards in life, such as painful thoughts, feelings, sensations, and memories, that can get in the way of chasing a life that matters, as well as the behaviors you do to try and escape, avoid, or control those experiences."

We may step back and ask participants what it feels like to look at this life map, or what they notice. End by explaining that focusing attention to notice what their behavior is about—whether it reflects them chasing a life that matters or an attempt to escape something painful—is the first practice for taking a more active role in life. They must notice what is happening before they can begin to make any changes. In one cohesive exercise, you have mapped the whole ACT model and demonstrated for participants a different way of viewing their life.

Life Map in Pairs

After completing the life map with the group, invite participants to pair up. Hand out one clipboard per pair, with two Mapping Your Life worksheets (Gordon & Borushok, 2017) and a pen attached to it, and then instruct them to use the worksheets to make a life map for one another. You can download the worksheet, along with other accessories for this book, at http://www.newharbinger.com/42358.

Allot each participant five to eight minutes to go through each of the guiding questions on the worksheet, getting to know their fellow participant and creating a map for them. Ring a bell when it's time for them to switch roles. You may want to walk around the room and check in with each pair to see how the exercise is going, and to offer assistance.

Group Dialogue: Debriefing the Life Map

Allow two to five minutes for eliciting feedback about how the exercise went. A favorite prompt of ours is "What did you notice?" The point is to use a completely open-ended prompt. Participants might say, "Wow! That was interesting," or "It's a lot of stuff I already know." Although in our experience the latter answer is rare, there's often a cynic in every group, and that's okay. The anticlimactic prompt of asking what was noticed is simply meant to socialize participants to paying attention and to the idea that there's no wrong answer. Sometimes a technical question comes up, such as "Now that we have this written out, we should just focus on the good and avoid the bad?" In such cases, we might playfully respond with this:

Well, that'd be ideal, but we don't make the map to avoid the nasty stuff. In my experience, we don't have control over it—it just keeps coming back.

Mapping Your Life

This is a map to your life. Following it is about paying attention to your experience so that you can choose what you do.

1. **Provide at least one answer for each section of your map.**

3. What do you do to escape, avoid, or control your painful experiences?

4. What would you choose to do or are you already doing to chase your values?

Me noticing

2. What painful thoughts, feelings, sensations, or memories get in the way of you chasing your values?

1. Who and what matter most to you? What qualities do you most wish to embody in your life? These are your personal values.

2. **Notice how your experiences are different by answering each question carefully.**

- What does it feel like to chase your values?

- What does it feel like to try and escape painful thoughts, feelings, sensations, and memories?

- Do you spend the majority of your life living your values or trying to escape painful experiences?

Instead, we're really focusing on paying attention to what we do in different situations, paying attention to how our behavior works when nasty stuff shows up, because that's what is going to empower us to be able to change—getting better at noticing.

Again and again, we bring participants back to the theme of this session: paying attention. It is the jumping-off point for all the work we do in the other sessions.

One last piece of advice. From time to time, we get a response like this from a participant: "I notice these things all the time." That's likely true, as sometimes folks who are distressed have a tendency to have hyperfocus or to analyze what they are experiencing as a way to control or avoid it. This is probably not the kind of noticing that we're promoting in this protocol, so we might respond like this:

> Great! Our challenge is to get you to pay attention to what you're doing at any given time in your life so that you're more aware of what's influencing your behavior, making it easier for you to choose what you do next. It's all a process of paying attention. As humans, we're not any good at ridding ourselves of the painful experiences we don't want. But if we pay attention to what we experience, we can begin to see how these experiences affect what we do—and that they don't have to. We can learn new ways to respond when they show up.

When wrapping up the discussion, we explain how the process of generating the life map and practicing yoga parallel each other. Noticing whether they're chasing their values or attempting to escape pain when building the life map is similar to intentionally being in the present moment while practicing yoga. It's all about noticing!

Yoga Is Paying Attention

You might transition into the yoga practice of the session with this script:

> In this practice, we're going to focus on sensory experiences of the body as a way to pay attention. Using the body and breath is a powerful way to train the mind to return to the present moment. Sensations that you feel in your body, like the movement of your breath, are experiences that are always available to you in the now. One of the wonderful things about the practice of yoga is that it doesn't ask you to do or be the impossible. It only invites you to be yourself—truly yourself, nothing extra. Our ability to tune in to our bodily sensations is the most immediate doorway into our moment-to-moment experience. Paying attention to them allows us to slow down and

really feel what we feel, to notice how the mind communicates ideas and theories about the experiences we're having. And then, to notice what we do next.

We find it helpful to tell participants that when we say "paying attention," we're not talking about some kind of hypervigilant awareness. Getting distracted from the body, getting wrapped up in thoughts, is not failure. In fact, in most instances, it is expected. It's simply part of the process of practicing paying attention, which is more about remembering and being willing to come back. You might share a story about when you found it difficult to pay attention, or examples of areas in life for which you struggle to be present. You might even share with participants how you often find your mind wandering during this practice, or even this session, but emphasize that the goal is to notice when our mind wanders and to then redirect our attention to the present.

You'll now conduct the first yoga sequence, composed of the following practices:

- Finding your seat and bringing attention to the breath

- Seated Sun Salutation

- Seated Side Angle

- Seated Cat

- Seated Cow

- Cow Face

- Seated Forward Fold

- Seated Twist

- Seated Vinyasa Flow

- Supported Lying Twist

Finding Your Seat and Bringing Attention to the Breath

Ask participants to find a stable posture, seated cross-legged or kneeling on the floor if possible, in which they can sit up straight. Sitting on a chair for this early practice is also okay. The most important principle here is to be seated as straight as possible while also avoiding rigidity in the posture or spine. For some, sitting on a pillow will lift the hips and tilt the pelvis forward, making this posture more accessible. If a pillow is not available, use a folded blanket. You can also invite participants to sit on the edge of a block, but this may be uncomfortable for longer periods of time.

Ask participants to rest their hands in their laps, forming a circle out of their hands, with thumbs touching and fingers overlapping. Have them slightly tuck the chin and lightly lift up through the crown of the head to help straighten and elongate the spine. Once everyone is seated as comfortably as possible, it's time to start the more formal practice.

Have participants take a breath on purpose, inhaling and letting out an exaggerated, audible sigh, perhaps with a sense of deep joy, if this is available to them. Alternatively, you may leave out the sigh and simply focus on breathing. Direct them to allow their eyes to relax. The eyes may close or remain open, whichever is most comfortable for them. Invite participants to bring their attention to the quality of their breath. "Can you breathe without being caught up in judgments?" They may notice judgments of themselves, their posture, their breath—anything really. The challenge here is to simply watch the breath.

Move into intentional breathing with long, full inhales and slow, controlled exhales. That being said, try not to make the goal about taking the deepest breath possible but instead the depth that feels appropriate. Deep breathing can inadvertently involve the upper shoulders and neck muscles (known as secondary accessory-musculature breathing). This type of breathing has the potential to overstimulate us because it simulates a sympathetic nervous system breath response. When someone is engaging in secondary accessory-musculature breathing, you might see the muscles in their neck tense or their shoulders begin to move, or both, neither of which is necessary for breathing. When someone continues to breathe in this way they may begin to experience a hyperaroused state that can induce an anxiety response.

You might use this script:

With an inhale, lift the shoulders up to the ears, gently squeeze the shoulders into a shrug, and make a fist with both hands. As you exhale, drop your shoulders and soften the hands.

Take a moment here to breathe and feel the sensations in the body. What was it like to tense up and release the tension from the body? Noticing if the movement helps or exacerbates any existing discomfort or pain.

With an inhale, lift the arms in front of the body, palms facing down. With an exhale, extend through the fingers, softening the shoulders. With an inhale, turn the palms facing up. With an exhale, turn the palms facing down. Repeat three more times.

Seated Sun Salutation (Floor Variation)

Have participants sit on the floor, if possible. Explain that they should sit with the spine active and erect but without creating rigidity in the posture. Sometimes we'll say, "Sit up with 75 percent of your maximum effort. That 25 percent of softness allows the breath to move in and out with ease." If sitting on the floor creates discomfort along the spine, in the hips, or around the knees, have participants experiment with sitting on a prop, such as a yoga block, a blanket, or a bolster. Biomechanically, this will allow the pelvis and the spine to naturally find a more neutral position. The prop helps the spine be tall without requiring as much effort to create tallness. Do this sequence twice.

Take a few moments here to connect with the sensation of the sit bones on the floor, perhaps rocking gently from side to side and sensing the breath moving through the body.

On an inhale, reach the arms up as you softly look toward the hands. As you look up, make sure you don't crane your neck too much, rather allow your eyes to do some of the work. On an exhale, fold forward from the hips, allowing the torso to fold over the thighs.

Placing the hands on the floor in front of you, inhale to lengthen up through the spine, drawing the shoulder blades back and opening the chest, creating a flat spine. Exhale as you fold the torso forward again over the thighs, allowing the spine to round slightly.

On an inhale, bring the torso back to an upright position as you reach the arms up, gazing toward the hands. Exhale to bring the hands to heart center [Añjali Mudrā], placing the palms together with the thumbs resting on the sternum [breastbone].

Seated Sun Salutation (Chair Variation)

Have participants start seated in a chair, sitting close to the edge, with feet flat on the floor and a little wider than the hips. If you notice participants with a rounded spine or pelvis tucked under them, have them try sitting on a blanket or two. Just like sitting on a block on the floor, the blankets raise the pelvis higher than the thigh bones, allowing the pelvis and spine to find a more neutral starting position with less effort. Once everyone is situated, take them through the pose twice.

Take a few moments here to really connect with the feeling of the sit bones on the chair, the feet on the floor, and the breath moving through the body.

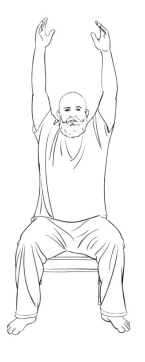

On an inhale, reach the arms up as you softly look toward the hands. Be sure not to crane your neck too much, rather allow your eyes to do some of the work.

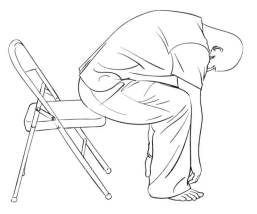

On an exhale, fold forward from the hips, allowing the torso to fall between the legs and letting the spine round.

If having the torso between the legs feels inappropriate for the hips or spine, keep the legs closer together and fold over the thighs.

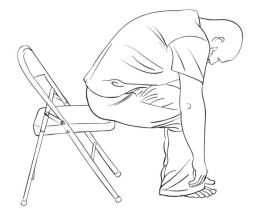

Placing the hands on the shins or knees, inhale to lengthen up through the spine, drawing the shoulder blades toward the spine and opening the chest to feel more broad across the collarbones.

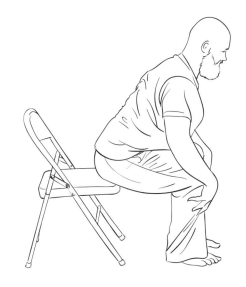

Exhale as you fold the torso forward again in between the legs or over the thighs, allowing the spine to round slightly. On an inhale, bring the torso back to an upright position as you reach the arms up, gazing toward the hands. Exhale to bring the hands to heart center [Añjali Mudrā]

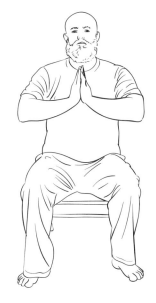

For a somewhat more advanced variation, after the first forward fold, rather than placing the hands on the shins, you could suggest that participants take the arms behind the back, interlacing the fingers. And as they inhale to lengthen the spine, have them reach the arms back and slightly up. This variation is in no way better, but if the back, core, and shoulders are feeling strong and open, it might be available to you and participants.

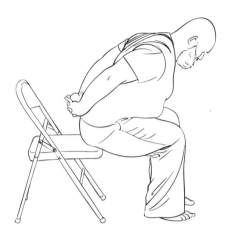

It is after this first sequence that we might ask participants to raise their hands if at some point they find themselves getting distracted by thoughts. We tend to raise our hands too. After some hands pop up, we'll usually respond with "Good noticing!" We explain that getting distracted by thinking is normal, and just like everyone else we, the facilitators, can get lost in thought even as our bodies and minds are performing tasks, such as teaching a yoga sequence. Remind them that the important part is to notice when their mind has wandered and to make a commitment to come back to the moment. This is the practice of mindfulness. This is the practice of dhāranā.

Seated Side Angle

With an inhale, lift up through the crown of the head. With an exhale, root down through the sit bones.

Inhale to reach both arms up. Exhale, bringing your right hand to the right side of the mat, or a block if mobility is limited, coming into a little side bend [lateral flexion]. You have the option to come down onto the elbow, if it is comfortable to do so. As you lean to one side, make sure that the spine does not rotate and the shoulders stay square.

Inhale to lift the gaze toward the left arm and move some breath into the left side of the rib cage. Exhale to settle more deeply into the pose.

Inhale to lift out of the pose using the right arm for some support and stability. Still inhaling, sweep the arms above the head, and lift the gaze. Exhale hands to heart center.

[*Repeat on the opposite side.*]

Seated Cat

This spinal flexion sequence can be done one to ten times.

On an inhale, bring hands in front of you, and interlace your fingers.

On an exhale, turn the palms to face away from you, pushing them away while rounding the spine, lightly scooping the pelvis into a posterior tilt, and tucking the chin. Feel the shoulder blades sliding away from the spine as you round.

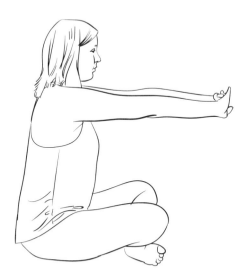

Inhale, release the hands, and, while sweeping the arms up in flexion, lift the gaze. Bring the head back if it feels appropriate.

Exhale to lower the hands to heart center, returning the spine to neutral.

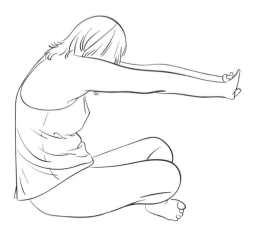

Seated Cow

This is a great pose for spinal extension. Feel free to move through this sequence one to ten times.

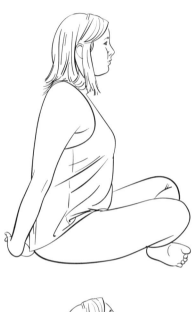

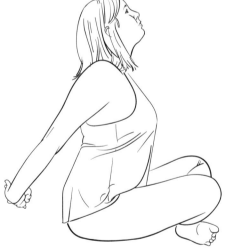

Inhale to draw the hands behind the back, interlacing the fingers.

Use the exhale to change the orientation of fingers, interlacing them opposite to what you did during Seated Cat. If the right pinky finger was on top, the left pinky finger should be on top this time.

Inhale to lift the arms. Engage the upper back to draw the shoulder blades into the spine, lifting the gaze and softly tilting the head back, broadening through the chest.

Exhale to release the hands. Inhale, sweeping the arms up in flexion and lifting the gaze. Bring the head back if it feels appropriate.

Exhale to release the hands to heart center.

Cow Face

Inhale, reaching through the crown of the head, and exhale, rooting down through the sit bones and finding a solid seat and long spine.

Inhale, reaching the right arm up. Exhale to bend the elbow, placing the right palm against the upper back, fingers reaching down toward the shoulder blade. The left hand comes behind the body, bending at the elbow as the left fingers reach for the right fingers. The back of the left hand will be in contact with the back. Clasp the fingers if possible, and inhale. [If the hands cannot touch or the shoulders are tight, participants can use a strap.] Avoid pushing the lower ribs or head forward. Soften the shoulders away from the ears without forcing them down.

Exhale to soften into the pose. Inhale into the ribs and up to the chest. On the next exhale, release the pose, coming back to center with a neutral spine and feeling the sensations in your body. [You can hold participants here anywhere from two to ten breaths.]

Feeling a stretching sensation is normal, but be aware of how the rest of the body and breath respond to those sensations. If the stretch is so intense that your body has to tighten up around it or the breath becomes rigid, you're stretching too far.

Inhale to sweep the arms up, and lift your gaze. Exhale hands to heart center.

Once you've completed the pose, have participants reverse how their legs are crossed. If the right leg is on top, have them put the left one on top, or vice versa. Then repeat the pose. Remind participants to, as always, be aware of their body. This side is different and may have more or less flexibility and strength. Remind them that they aren't striving for symmetry, especially at the risk of strain or injury.

Seated Forward Fold

Inhale to reach up through the crown of the head and root down through the sit bones, buttocks, or whatever part of your body is making contact with the mat. Exhale to hinge at the hips, folding forward while maintaining length in the spine. Still exhaling, gently reach the arms forward and extend the fingers to the floor. [Generally, we suggest that rather than straining to get the hands to the floor, participants should bring the floor to them by placing their hands on blocks.]

Inhale to fill the lungs. Tuck the chin and exhale deeper into the pose, lengthening through the back of the spine.

Inhale, pushing through the hands into the floor for assistance, slowly coming out of the forward fold. Come back to a seated position, reaching through the crown of the head, spine straight.

An option in this movement is to add a slight rounding to the spine as you exhale, like the Seated Cat movement. This degree of rounding, however, is contraindicated for individuals experiencing certain physical conditions, such as bulging or ruptured spinal discs or sciatica.

Seated Twist

On an inhale, reach the right arm behind the body, pressing the hand into the mat. Preferably, the right hand is aligned behind the right buttock.

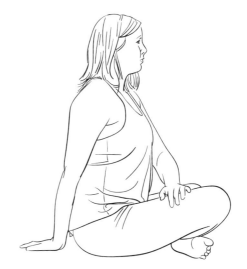

If you have to lean back to reach the floor, it's better to bring the floor up to you by placing the hand on a block or folded blanket.

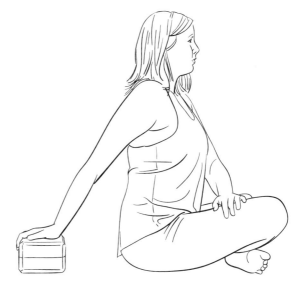

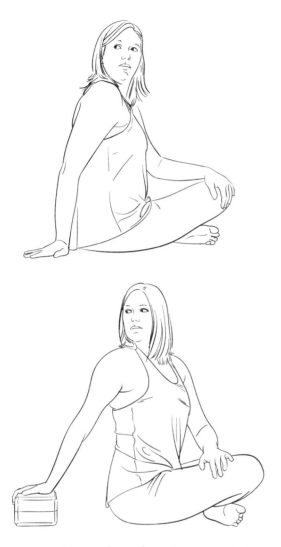

Reach the left hand to the right thigh. Lightly rock the pelvis forward to help lengthen the spine. Exhale to twist right. Begin by turning the low spine, then the upper spine and shoulders, then the head, and finally, the eyes look right.

With every inhale, lightly lift through the sternum, using the push of the right hand to assist. With every exhale, deepen the twist as much as is comfortably available. [We usually ask participants to notice the tendency to want to use the strength of the arms to force the twist deeper, encouraging them to notice any thoughts that arise and maybe even easing back a bit.]

As you twist, try to feel that the muscle of the side waist, or the obliques, and the musculature along the spine are twisting you, and that the arms are only there to aid in the twist. [Sometimes we'll say that if the obliques are the CEO of a twist, the arms are there to make copies and get lattes. They are a valuable part of the team but shouldn't be running the show. You can hold participants here from two to ten breaths.]

Inhale to release the head, slowly untwist back to center, and release the right and then left arm. [A really nice way to feel the release is to ask students to feel for the chin coming back in line with the chest, the chest coming back in line with the belly button, and finally the belly button coming back in line with the pelvis.] Inhale to sweep the arms up, lifting the gaze. Exhale hands to heart center.

[*Repeat for the opposite side of the body.*]

Seated Vinyasa Flow

It is now time to turn the yoga practice into a flow, in which one pose transitions into the next smoothly, like a dance. The breath is an important component of this practice, so be sure to clearly instruct participants for when they should inhale and exhale. Encourage participants to move at their own pace, using the full length of inhalations and exhalations for transitions between poses. Also, reinforce that the goal is not to keep up with others but instead to practice the dance at a pace that is appropriate for them. A cue to notice how the body feels as it flows from one pose to the next may help bring participants back into the moment, if their minds have wandered. You may cue them to notice sensations or what their minds say about their practice or abilities.

Beginning from a seated position, inhale to sweep the arms up, and lift the gaze. Exhale hands to heart center. Inhale to sweep the arms up, and lift the gaze. Exhale hands down on the floor in front of you, and hinge at the hips to fold all the way forward into a Seated Forward Fold. Inhale to rest, and exhale to soften more deeply into the pose. Inhale to lift back up to center, reaching the arms up and lifting the gaze. Exhale hands to heart center.

Inhale hands forward, interlacing the fingers with palms facing out. On the exhale, roll through the spine to Seated Cat.

Inhale to return to center, and exhale to release the arms.

Inhale to sweep the arms up, and lift the gaze. Exhale hands to heart center.

Inhale to sweep the arms up. Exhale to bring the arms down and behind the back, interlacing the opposite fingers.

Inhale to reach back with the arms, broadening through the chest in Seated Cow. Exhale to release the posture, bringing hands to your sides.

Inhale to sweep both arms up. Exhale the right hand to the right side of the mat for Seated Side Angle, coming down onto the elbow if it is comfortable. Inhale to lift the gaze to the left arm, breathing into the left side of the ribs. Exhale to settle more deeply into the pose.

Inhale back to a tall, vertical spine, and sweep the arms up, lifting the gaze. Exhale the hands down and hinge at the hips to fold forward into a Seated Forward Fold.

Inhale back to vertical, reaching the arms up. Exhale the left hand to the left side of the mat, coming down onto the elbow if it is comfortable. Inhale to lift the gaze to the right arm, breathing into the right side of the ribs. Exhale to settle more deeply into the pose.

Inhale to sweep the arms up, lifting the gaze with a tall spine. Exhale hands down and hinge at the hips to fold forward in Seated Forward Fold.

Inhale back to vertical, reaching the arms up. Exhale hands to heart center.

Change the legs to the opposite cross.

Inhale to sweep the arms up, lifting the gaze. Exhale hands to heart center.

Inhale to place the right hand behind the back, left hand to the right knee. Exhale to a Seated Twist, beginning with the torso, then the head, and finally the eyes looking to the right. Inhale to lift the sternum, reaching through the crown of the head, stretching through the spine. Exhale to deepen the twist, looking farther with the eyes.

Inhale to lift, and exhale to return to center with a neutral spine.

Inhale to sweep the arms up, lifting the gaze. Exhale hands to heart center.

Inhale to place the left hand behind the back, right hand to the left knee. Exhale to a Seated Twist, beginning with the torso, then the head, and finally the eyes looking to the left. Inhale to lift the sternum, reaching through the crown of the head, stretching through the spine. Exhale to twist deeper, looking farther with the eyes.

Inhale to lift, and exhale to return to center, untwisting the body to a neutral position.

Inhale to sweep the arms up, lifting the gaze. Exhale the hands down and hinge at the hips to fold all the way forward into Seated Forward Fold. Inhale here to rest, and exhale to soften more deeply into the pose.

Inhale to come back to center. Exhale to release the breath.

Inhale to sweep the arms up, lifting the gaze. Exhale hands to heart center, softly pushing them into one another, feeling the opposing action. Close your eyes.

Have participants remain here for several breaths, with eyes closed. Invite them to notice and take stock of what they're feeling.

Supported Lying Twist

In the ayurvedic model of physiology, twisting positions are seen as *adaptogenic*, meaning they balance the nervous system. This makes them ideal for slowing and cooling down at the end of a yoga sequence or for when one is anxious or on edge. Twists can also work to counteract tiredness, fatigue, or sluggishness by helping to create more of a soft alertness in the mind.

Lie down on your back with legs out straight. Draw the right knee into the chest, holding the leg in place with the hands around the right knee. Keeping the left hand on the right knee, place the right arm off to the side straight out from the shoulder, resting the arm on the floor. Actively but not aggressively press the right shoulder down into the mat. Keeping the right shoulder down, move the right leg across the midline of the body toward the left, coming into a twisted position. If the right knee can't come to the floor without the right shoulder lifting, place props under the right leg for support. Turn your head to the right.

It is really important to let go of the idea that the deeper the twist, the more successful the position. You might find that even though there is a large range of motion available, not all of that range feels comfortable, and some of it might even be painful. It is important that the body is not in pain or overly uncomfortable in this posture or any other.

After a few breaths, you might notice the body begin to soften more deeply into the posture. This is an invitation for one of two things: either to stay and simply enjoy the softness or to remove or adjust the prop under the right leg. If you remove or adjust the prop, just be aware of how the body responds, especially if an uncomfortable or painful sensation arises. We are not trying to convince ourselves that we're comfortable if we're not. There is always the option to put the prop back.

Repeat the posture on the other side. As participants move their props to the opposite side of the mat, prompt them to stay with their breath, making the act of switching props a part of the practice.

Group Dialogue: Debriefing Yoga Practice

After participants come out of their twist, the facilitator should positively reinforce the group's participation, announcing that they just completed their first yoga practice. Tim tends to do this with a smile and in a loud, celebratory manner, whereas Steve is a little more subdued. Overall, you want to create an encouraging and congratulatory atmosphere. Even being in a room with other people and doing these physical movements may have been an extraordinary act of courage, especially for those who truly followed the prompts to listen to their body, modifying poses to fit their needs and abilities.

Hopefully you noticed that we didn't simply use stereotypical yoga cues or canned lessons. Rather, throughout the practice, we reinforced the need for participants to identify the difference between moving toward values and trying to escape painful experiences. This group dialogue is an opportunity for you, the facilitator, to make explicit this discrimination task and to invite reflections from participants.

You may ask, "Did anyone notice themselves wanting to go to their happy place or forcing themselves to do a pose or movement that didn't feel right?" A participant answering yes to either question is not problematic. Remember, the core of this work is having participants pay attention on purpose to their behavior. It's a good thing if they noticed this!

Sweet Spot

This exercise is an adaptation of Wilson's (2009) sweet spot exercise that brings together all six of ACT's processes and has an evocative element of perspective taking involved. We invite participants to break back into their pairs, explaining:

> We're going to do a brief eyes-closed meditation on something sweet from our life. We will open our eyes to continue the meditation, sharing our sweet thing with one another. We won't be sharing why that moment was sweet, but instead we'll focus on what we noticed in that sweet moment. We won't be pausing to debrief the experience between turns; rather we'll continue to sit in this meditation with one another.

Some participants may not be comfortable engaging in this exercise, so address this at the outset: "Remember, if you don't wish to participate and would feel more comfortable sitting back and watching the group process, I'll ask you to check if that's a move toward your values or away from pain. I'll support you in whatever you choose to do." Then, have participants sit across from their partner, and begin the meditation.

> If it is comfortable for you, allow your eyes to close or lower your gaze and allow your vision to soften its focus. Take a breath on purpose.

Notice the sensations of breathing, how the belly expands on the inhale and collapses on the exhale. Inevitably distractions arise, whether they're sensations, thoughts, feelings, or memories. Whatever shows up, breathe it in. Notice it on purpose. Exhale and come right back to the breath.

Imagine that your history is stretched out before you, that you can reach back throughout your life to different moments. Bring your attention to a moment that is of some sweetness for you, however small or seemingly insignificant it may seem. It could be something as simple as waking up before everyone else in the house and getting to use all the hot water in the shower, or a recent cup of coffee or tea that you really savored, perhaps for its flavor and warmth against your hand. Whatever moment of sweetness occurs to you, pause there. Take a breath and really breathe in the moment.

Allow yourself to be there behind your eyes, remembering the details, including the colors, shapes, and textures you saw and the sounds you heard. Really be there. Notice what it was like to be in that moment. If your mind skips ahead to a different moment, let that be okay. Just take a breath, inhale, and come back to your moment of sweetness, like hitting the instant-replay button. Alternatively, if some bitterness shows up in that moment of sweetness, such as a sense of loss because someone in that moment is no longer in your life, just pause and notice that too.

In a moment's time, I'm going to invite you to open your eyes, and without any negotiation, one of you will begin to share your moment of sweetness. Describe the sensory details, what it was like to be there. What shapes, colors, or textures did you notice? What did you hear? Your mind is going to want to explain why that moment was significant or give backstory, but see if you can let that go and just allow this person who is listening to hear the moment. And if you find yourself in the position of listening, just allow yourself to be present to this other human being, sharing a moment of sweetness. Notice your impulse to nod your head, to want to ask questions, make comments, or engage in other active listening. If the person sharing their moment has seemingly finished, notice your impulse to fill the silence or to share your moment. Don't worry, I will guide you in what to do next, but just pause in that silence together until we move on as a group.

In your own time, allow your eyes to open. Notice the face of the person sitting across from you. Without negotiation, one of you begin sharing your moment of sweetness. [Generally we ring a bell or sound a singing bowl after one to two minutes to signal the group to come to silence.]

Coming to silence, allowing your eyes to close or your vision to soften its focus. Take a breath on purpose and notice whatever you may be feeling right now. If you were the one sharing, what was it like for you to allow this other person into your world, to see that moment of sweetness from behind your eyes? And if you were the one listening, what was it like for you to show up to this person's moment? What could it have meant to them that you allowed yourself to just take them in, to be a witness to something sweet in their life?

Taking a breath here on purpose, notice anything that shows up for you. And prepare yourself to switch roles. If you were the one sharing, you will now be listening, and if you were the one who was just listening, you will now be the one sharing. Take a breath, and return to your moment of sweetness, remembering what it was like to be there behind your eyes, noticing the sensory details: what you heard, the shapes or colors you noticed. Your mind is going to want to explain why the moment was sweet, give the backstory, but just allow this person sitting across from you to be in that experience with you, as if they could be there behind your eyes, seeing what you saw, hearing what you heard.

Inhale on purpose, feeling the belly expand. Exhale, noticing the chest drop as the belly collapses, pushing air out of your body. On your next inhale, opening your eyes, and in your own time sharing your moment of sweetness. [Again, we generally allow one to two minutes—the same amount as earlier—before signaling the end of this exchange.]

Coming to silence, allow your eyes to close or to soften their focus. Take a breath on purpose and notice whatever feeling shows up for you in this moment. If you were the one sharing your moment of sweetness, what was it like for you to allow your partner into your world, to see that moment of sweetness from behind your eyes? And if you were the one listening, what was it like for you to hear that moment of sweetness? And if your mind is coming up with some kind of judgment, like *Shit, they picked their kids—I should've picked mine. They're going to think I'm a bad parent.* Just notice that, breathe it in, and come back to being here now, in this moment. Could you go behind their eyes and see what they saw, hear what they heard, feel what they felt? What could it have meant to them that you allowed yourself to just take them in, to be a witness to something sweet in their life?

One last time, let's take a breath on purpose, have an extralong inhale, and really feel the belly expand. Exhale all the way out to feel the belly collapse. On your next inhale, open your eyes. Take a moment here to notice the face of the person sitting across from you, to notice their eyes, the features of their face. In a way that feels respectful, take a moment to thank them for doing this exercise with you, for journeying down a path of vulnerability with you.

Group Dialogue: Debriefing the Sweet Spot

Allow two to five minutes for eliciting feedback about how the exercise went. Our favorite prompt is "What did you notice during that exercise?" Participants may comment that they were surprised by how intensely they felt the sweet moment, while others may comment that they felt uncomfortable or vulnerable sharing. As the listener, participants may notice how difficult it was not to respond or to reassure the other person who was sharing. This is a great exercise in perspective taking, as well as for sitting in the present moment. It's easy to turn to explaining a memory, but it is much harder as both the speaker and listener to simply experience or witness it. This exercise highlights how easy it is to be caught up in language and to miss the actual moment because it forces people to interact with each other and with themselves in a new way.

Session One Home Practice: A Bold Move

The work participants do in session is a mirror of the behaviors and processes we are encouraging out of session, and therefore their work does not end when the session does. Each week, participants will have a home practice to complete. This provides them an opportunity outside the yoga studio or therapy group room to bring to life in a concrete, actionable way some of the abstract principles we're teaching through MYACT. Our hope is that participants will go home and use what we have done in the group.

Invite participants to pair up one last time for this session. Give them two minutes each to describe a single action they can engage in today that will move them boldly toward who and what matter most to them. While still in pairs, give each participant two minutes to describe an obstacle, be it a thought, feeling, sensation, or memory, that might get in the way of them making their bold move. Instruct participants to finish each exchange by telling their partner that they support them in moving toward their values. We also encourage participants to use the Mapping Your Life worksheet at home with someone they care about, making a life map for them.

Ending Savasana: Body Scan

Savasana, also known as Corpse Pose or Dead Body Pose, is how we end every yoga practice in this manual. Please note that this Savasana practice may not work for some populations. For example, getting in touch with bodily sensations may be distressing for trauma survivors with severe dissociative issues. Alternatively, people suffering with chronic pain issues may have difficulty lying on their back. If you're working with such individuals, you might instead use a slow moving meditation, or you might use Savasana without the body scan element. We also highly recommend that participants use pillows, blankets, and bolsters to support them in this passive posture.

Invite participants to lie down with their head at the top of their mat, feet pointed away from the group. Turn the lights down, if possible, but not off. Invite them to relax their eyelids. The eyes may close or remain open. Ask them to extend their legs and arms. Their feet should flop open, with toes pointing in opposite directions. If low back pain is an issue, invite participants to place the soles of their feet flat on the mat with knees bent. The knees will lean into one another for support. Arms should be extended along the sides of the body, palms face up. Participants may wish to sit on a chair or on their mat with their back supported if they experience mobility issues.

Today I invite you to do a body scan exercise with me in which we will practice noticing the sensations happening within our own body. You may find that you notice areas of tension or relaxation that you weren't aware of, or you may find yourself not wanting to pay attention to certain parts of your body that bring you pain. These are all normal experiences. I ask that in serving your own progress, and in developing your own practice of awareness, that you try your best to notice all of your experiences during this exercise, even those you don't want.

This practice doesn't ask you to feel less tense, nor is there any expectation or desired outcome. Instead, let go of making goals for yourself during this practice. Let go of judgmental or critical thoughts. Give yourself permission to feel what you're feeling right now and to make space for everything that shows up.

If it feels comfortable, please allow your eyes to close gently, or simply allow them to gaze softly at the ceiling.

If you find your mind wandering, traveling to the past or future or a "what if" scenario, or making noise and commenting on the exercise, simply notice where your mind is taking you. Listen to the noise, acknowledge it, and bring yourself back to the sound of my voice and the part of your body I am directing your attention to.

Begin by bringing your attention to your breath, to the fact that you're breathing. Noticing the rise and fall of your chest and belly as you breathe in and out… Try not to manipulate your breath in any way. Simply observe the breath. Your natural way of breathing… Throughout this exercise, you may notice a resistance to doing something that I invite you to do. Remember to always choose what is best for you. You always have the option of returning to the breath, breathing deep into the belly.

Now gently turn your attention to the top of your head. Notice if you can feel the area just above your head, paying attention to any sensation of warmth or coolness… Start here and gently, slowly turn your mind's eye inward and begin to scan down your body. Noticing all the tiny muscles in your face. Can you feel any of them tightening or loosening with relaxation?

Can you feel the cool air enter your nostrils and the warm air exhaling through the nose as you breathe? Continuing down to the positioning of your tongue in your mouth, noticing saliva in your mouth begin to pool as you pay attention, the feel of your tongue in your mouth as you swallow.

Next, lowering your mind's eye to the point where your neck meets your head…and slowly scanning down to the point where your neck meets the rest of your body…paying attention to the sensations there and expanding your awareness to any thoughts or feelings that may arise as you scan down to your shoulders. Breathe into those thoughts and feelings, and with an exhale, follow your attention down your shoulders. if you feel comfortable, bring your shoulders up to your ears and then gently roll them back and down, noticing any change in sensation with the movement… Slowly draw your attention down your shoulders to the tips of your fingers… Can you feel the point where your fingers end and the air begins?

If you notice that your mind has begun to wander, that's alright. That's what minds do. Simply acknowledge where your mind has gone and bring your attention back to the sound of my voice and the part of your body I am directing your attention to.

Turning your attention to your back, noticing your posture and following the curve of your spine…feeling the points where your back touches the chair… Slowly wrap your attention around to your stomach, feeling how the abdomen expands with an in-breath and deflates with an out-breath… moving down to your hips, feeling the weight of your body sitting in the chair, the places where your legs meet the chair…noticing any sensations as you move down your thighs, around your knees, to the backs of your legs, and finally to your feet… Can you feel any sensation from the soles of your feet? Maybe wiggle your toes. Can you feel each individual toe? Do you feel any sensation of warmth or coolness?

Gently draw your attention back up your body to your chest and belly, feeling as they expand and deflate with each inhale and exhale…noticing with curiosity if your breathing has changed at all from the beginning of this exercise…noticing your own practice of noticing throughout this exercise.

Begin to turn your attention away from your body to the room around you. Listening to the sound of your breath, and to the sounds around you both soft and loud, and near or far away…listening to the sound of my voice as I walk you through this exercise… And in your own time, when you are ready, gently fluttering your eyes open or raising your head.

In your own time rolling to the right side and using your left arm to support you in lifting yourself out of this pose. We will finish our work together today seated at the front of our mats as we begin our good-bye ritual.

Ending with Chanting

With all of the participants out of Savasana and seated at the front of their mats, invite them to chant "Om" three times in a row. In our experience, it's helpful to explain that "Om" represents all things that have happened, are happening, and ever will happen. When chanting "Om," we hold space for all of those things in our minds and hearts.

Explain that no special note or tone is required for chanting. The only instruction is that each participant chants "Om" for the full length of their exhale. Participants don't need to start or end at the same time as the rest of the participants.

Sharing Appreciations

At the conclusion of the chanting, invite each participant to share something they have appreciated about their first MYACT session: "In just a few words, could you please share what you appreciated about our session today? It could be about something we did together, something someone else did that touched your heart, something you did, or something you experienced."

For sessions with cofacilitators, it's helpful to begin this process with one of the facilitators modeling what sharing an appreciation is like. Then have each participant share an appreciation before finishing with the other facilitator. When the group is shy and there is only one facilitator, the facilitator should begin by sharing an appreciation. However, when possible, we recommend that the facilitator shares their appreciation last.

Closing Posture

From a seated position at the front of your mat (or seated on a chair), place your hands at heart center, invite participants to place their hands similarly, and explain, "You may have heard the word 'namaste.' It's often used to greet or end an interaction. We'll use the word with the hands at heart center. Like 'savasana' and 'yoga,' 'namaste' is Sanskrit. It means 'The light in me recognizes and bows to the light in you.'

Then, bow your head, touch your thumbs (pressed together in Añjali Mudrā) between the eyebrows (the third eye), and say "namaste" aloud while bowing your upper body forward.

Working with Individuals

If you're using MYACT with an individual client, here are some modifications you might make to the way you deliver session one.

- Shorten the orientation and introduction to fit your practice setting.

- The beginning and ending Savasana could be done in a chair as an eyes-closed meditation, if desired.

- The group life map and life map in pairs should be condensed to facilitate a life map with the individual. We recommend trying to get multiple responses for each quadrant.

- If you are in a direct practice setting, you may choose to shorten the yoga practice to include only the seated postures in a chair, but don't be afraid to move the furniture and get on a mat. That's what we do.

- During the sweet spot exercise, only the client should share a sweet moment. This exercise can be done as more of a conversation. Prompt the client to describe what they experienced in the moment they're describing rather than falling back on explaining. If functionally appropriate, you can share your response to hearing their sweet moment or share your own sweet moment, or both.

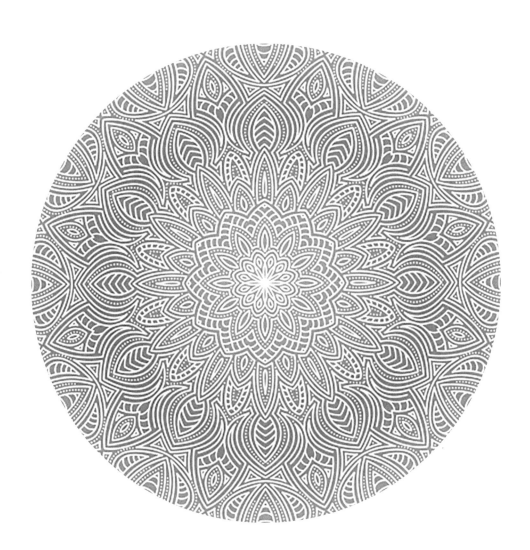

Samskāra

The second session of MYACT advances the dhāranā practice of noticing from session one and focuses more explicitly on tracking *outcomes*, what participants do when their painful experiences show up. In the Yoga Sūtras, these patterns of responding are called *samskāras*. Through identifying and observing these patterns, participants are exposed to the unworkable reactions that occur when they take painful private experiences literally. They begin to see the function of their behaviors in terms of both short- and long-term outcomes.

Throughout this session, defusion is used with present-moment processes to encourage participants to be aware of experiences that influence their behavior. Conceptually, we find that participants get stuck on rigid rules about painful experiences. For example, "I won't react with hostility toward my brother-in-law as soon as he isn't an asshole!" We don't debate the merits or deficiencies of the brother-in-law. He may very well be an asshole. Instead, we come back to the participant's experience of the brother in-law. With curiosity, we inquire which thoughts, feelings, sensations, or memories show up for this participant, helping them label the private experience explicitly so they can notice it and choose what they want to do next.

Beginning Meditation: The Two Yous

You may need to remind participants to start the session in silence, positioning themselves in Savasana or a different passive posture that is appropriate for them. We find it helpful to remind the first few participants who enter the group space to begin in this way. The room should be set in such a way that it stimulates participants to enter in silence and position themselves silently in a relaxation posture. We tend to have the lights dimmed, and either soft music is playing or the room is silent.

This beginning meditation encourages participants to observe two different ways of being in the world. Invite them to practice present-moment awareness. You'll use that awareness to help them make contact with their values and later to draw a distinction between two forms of behavior: a life governed by painful private experiences and one led by a connection to values. This exercise focuses on defusion and values processes by bringing participants' awareness to a version of themselves reacting to painful private experiences in one instance, and then, from another perspective, picturing themselves acting on their values, living the qualities they find important.

Welcome to the second session of MYACT. Find yourself in any relaxation pose that works for you, seated or flat on your back. If you require assistance, please raise a hand. If you're experiencing low back pain today, you may wish to sit upright or to lie down with feet flat on the floor and knees bent. If lying in Savasana, position your arms out to the sides of your body, palms facing up, feet splayed out. Take a breath here on purpose, and notice the sensations of breathing in your body.

In this practice, I'm going to guide you to bring attention to different areas of your life. If you find yourself distracted, take a breath, notice your distractions, and come back to the instructions. Let's begin with our practice.

Breathing here, notice the sensations of breathing in your body, noticing how the belly expands on an inhale and collapses on an exhale.

Really stay with the movement of breath in your body. Inevitably, distractions arise. Your job is not to avoid distractions but to notice them. You will have distractions. Take a breath on purpose when you notice distractions, and come back to the movement of your breath.

I'd like to invite you to picture yourself interacting with someone who's important to you, maybe at work, at school, while volunteering, or at home. Imagine yourself with this person, and imagine you're being pushed around by some thoughts. Really see yourself hooked by your thoughts. How do you react to them? How might you behave in this moment? What is the look on your face? See yourself there with that look. And what does the tone of your voice sound like? What does the posture of your body look like? Really see yourself in this state of mind, reacting to painful thoughts, feelings, sensations, or memories, and see how this reactive state impacts your behavior. Really picture yourself there. Take a breath and notice what it feels like to observe this version of you, to see your reactive, hooked self.

Let's go ahead and come back to the present moment. Breathing, letting go of the image of your reactive self. Take a breath and notice the sensations of breathing in your body.

I'm now going to invite you to picture yourself again interacting with someone who's important to you, at work, at school, from volunteering, or at home. But this time, I'm going to invite you to imagine yourself connected with what is important to you, acting on those values and qualities that you want to be about. Really see yourself living those qualities that matter most to you. What does your face look like? What is the look in your eyes in that moment? What does your posture look like? Really see yourself there and breathe it in. This is a version of yourself who is deeply connected to these areas of your life that you wish to connect with more deeply and grow your behavior toward.

What is it like here to observe this version of you? Take a breath here and notice how that feels. And allowing that image to pass as you come back to this present moment. Feeling the sensations of the chair you're sitting on supporting your body. Noticing sensations of the breath. When you're ready, bringing some motion into the body, whether it's a wiggle of the fingers, a rotation of the wrists, a rolling of the shoulders up, forward, and down, or a gentle motion to the neck as you turn the head from side to side.

Coming back to this room, opening your eyes. If you're on your back, roll to your right and use your left arm to prop yourself up and come to a seated position.

Looking around, noticing the other participants here in this room, and seeing people who also have thoughts, feelings, sensations, and memories that push them around.

Group Dialogue: Debriefing Beginning Meditation

Take a breath, and in silence, look at each participant, perhaps making eye contact, smiling, nodding, or otherwise acknowledging them. Do a visual check-in. Then break the silence by asking, "What did you notice in that meditation?" and engage in a dialogue with the participants.

Group Dialogue: Debriefing Home Practice

The debriefing of home practice is an opportunity to talk about how participants fared with it, to reinforce their engagement in new behaviors, and to also troubleshoot problems that may have arisen.

Take ten minutes to first check in and ask each participant to share something about their experience of bringing MYACT home with them. Ask if they noticed moments during the week when they found themselves moving away from a painful private experience, attempting to control, avoid, or escape something they didn't want to feel, and times when they were moving toward who and what are most important to them, acting on a value. Be sure to check in about the "bold move" they shared in the previous session. During this discussion, you should also share your own experiences, both to model appropriate behavior and to enliven the conversation and set the right tone—that is, all sharing and vulnerability are welcome. Here are some prompts you might want to use:

Before we move on, how did everyone feel after they went home last week?

Did you have difficulties or successes with the home practice?

How was it to do this practice or to not do it?

What was it like to do the bold move?

Were there any barriers to doing it?

What did you notice while doing it?

> **Pro Tip:** Participants may feel compelled to lie about their bold move if they didn't do it, or they may be hesitant to share that they didn't do it. This helps no one. When reflecting on the home practice, it may be helpful to state in advance that some people may not have completed their bold move, and that it's okay. In fact, the lack of completion is a great opportunity for participants to notice what showed up and got in the way. You may even refer back to the life map to help facilitate that discussion: "What showed up that made it difficult for you to engage in your bold move? When that painful thought, feeling, sensation, or memory showed up, how did you respond to it?" You may even want to praise their good noticing as a way to reinforce their honesty and openness with the group.

Noticing Struggles

End the debriefing by facilitating a group discussion in which participants share difficult thoughts or feelings that they've struggled with. This is a good time for facilitators to self-disclose a personal struggle. For example, some may feel like an imposter, think *I'm not a very good facilitator or yoga teacher*, worry about not having something clever or sophisticated to say in session, or wonder if participants think they're not intelligent or qualified enough to treat them.

Ask participants how often they have these thoughts or feelings, emphasizing that many people experience similar thoughts and feelings regularly. When someone shares a painful struggle, normalize the experience by asking the group, "Can anyone else relate to this? Have other people also felt this way?"

Group Life Map: Looking for Stuck Patterns

We return to the group life map in session two to demonstrate how participants can get stuck in behavior patterns, avoiding one private experience only to reinforce yet another painful experience with little positive long-term effects. You should conduct a functional analysis of the group's life map and encourage participants to break into groups of two and identify stuck behavior patterns in their life maps.

Functional Analysis of the Group Life Map

Using a whiteboard, chalkboard, flip chart, or projector, re-create the group life map from session one. You should have it prepared before the session begins.

Explain the life map briefly, pointing to each quadrant and reminding readers of what they represent:

The bottom-right quadrant is about living the life that matters to us.

The bottom-left quadrant is what we don't want to feel.

The top-left quadrant is what we do to try and escape the things we don't want to feel.

The top-right quadrant is what we do to pursue the life that matters to us.

Now, rate the short-term and long-term impacts of the behaviors listed in the top-left quadrant. It doesn't matter whether the behavior seems adaptive or maladaptive. Our task here is to simply track how effective each behavior is for escaping painful thoughts, feelings, sensations, or memories. For each behavior, ask the group, "Does the behavior help you escape painful experiences in the moment?" You can indicate a yes with a checkmark and a no with an *X*. After you've completed that, repeat the process by asking, "Does the behavior permanently alleviate or remove the experience?" Again, note the yes or no answers with the marks of your choosing.

> **Pro Tip:** Participants may be confused by the prompt "Does the behavior permanently alleviate or remove the experience?" You can follow up by asking, "Has doing this [*point to a behavior in the top-left quadrant*] ever permanently deleted this [*point to an experience in the bottom-left quadrant*] so that now you no longer experience it?" The answer is always no. The point you want to highlight with this exercise is that certain behaviors may make a painful thought, feeling, sensation, or memory go away for a little while, but eventually, it always comes back. Trying to escape, avoid, or control painful private experiences doesn't actually work.

Now, ask participants if each behavior helps to bring them closer to who and what are most important to them. Indicate a yes or no with checkmarks or *X*'s, respectively, or whatever marks you choose. Participants will likely answer no to the majority of the behaviors because often they are not what they want to be doing when pain shows up—sometimes quite the opposite!

Feeling Stuck?

Show participants how trying to escape (behavior, top-left quadrant) a painful experience (bottom-left quadrant) can actually lead to more painful experiences (bottom-left quadrant) and more escape behaviors (top-left quadrant). See if you can connect three, four, five, or even six of these escape behaviors to painful thoughts, feelings, sensations, or memories. The exchange may look something like this:

Facilitator: So let's see how this plays out in real life. What is one thing down here [*pointing to bottom-left quadrant*] that usually shows up for someone?

Participant: Frustration with my husband for not doing whatever chore I asked him to do.

Facilitator: So when frustration shows up, what do you do in response?

Participant: I begin to think about all the different times he hasn't done what I asked.

Facilitator: Okay, so you start to ruminate. How do you feel afterward? [*Draws a line from "frustration" to "ruminate/think of past memories" in the top-left quadrant.*]

Participant: [*Laughs.*] More frustrated.

Facilitator: [*Chuckles.*] I can totally see that it just gets you more worked up. [*Draws a line from "ruminate/think of past memories" back down to "frustration."*] What happens next?

Participant: I ignore him when he tries to talk to me.

Facilitator: Hmm. So maybe he's trying to ask you about your day or what you want to have for dinner and you either don't respond or give one-word answers? [*Draws a line from "frustration" to "ignore him" in the top-left quadrant.*] Is the frustration gone?

Participant: No, then I feel frustrated *and* annoyed that he doesn't know why I'm upset.

Facilitator: So not only are you really frustrated but you're annoyed and thinking to yourself, *Oh my god! Can't he see I'm upset? Why doesn't he get why I'm pissed?* [*Points to other private experiences or writes in new ones.*] Then what happens?

Participant: I yell at him, and then I feel awful for exploding.

Facilitator: So all of this frustration and annoyance, and thinking *Why doesn't he realize what's bothering me?*, builds until you end up yelling, but then it sounds like immediately afterward you feel bad for yelling at him. [*Draws a line from "frustration/annoyance/thought" in the bottom-left quadrant to "yelling" in the top-left quadrant back down to "awful/bad."*] Can you see how this one attempt to escape frustration sucked you into this big avoidance loop?

Participant: Yeah, that's what always happens, and I hate it.

Finish the exchange by explaining that this is what we call being stuck:

This pattern makes perfect sense, because escaping what we don't want to feel generally works in the short term, which is why we keep avoiding certain experiences. The problem is that we learn a dangerous lesson: escaping what we don't want to feel is a viable way of working with our pain. We have to be sensitive and notice when a behavior isn't working in the long term, when it gets in the way of us connecting with who and what matter most to us.

Good or Bad, It Doesn't Matter

Take a moment to reiterate to participants that escaping what they don't want to feel isn't inherently bad. It can actually be a good thing: "Look, escaping painful experiences isn't all bad. If a bus careens toward you when you leave the group today, I want you to MOVE OUT OF ITS WAY!!! This group is about getting better at paying attention to how our behavior works in different situations, noticing what motivates our behavior."

Finish by asking participants to share examples of their own stuck patterns they can identify.

Stuck Patterns in Pairs

Have the group break into pairs:

Go ahead and break back into your groups of two and exchange your life maps from the previous session with each other. Go through your partner's life map, looking at and asking about how your partner's escape behaviors are working in the short term and long term. Are these behaviors moving them closer to the type of life they want to have? See if you can notice any patterns in which one painful experience leads to an escape behavior, and that attempt to escape, avoid, or control leads to more painful thoughts, feelings, sensations, or memories. This should be a conversation. One person will go first, asking questions of the other, and then you'll switch roles.

We tend to transition participants into their pairs with a lighthearted comment, such as "Yes, this means we're focusing on problematic behaviors for now, but, hey, we didn't come here without difficulties, right? If so, you might be in the wrong yoga class!"

Group Dialogue: Debriefing Stuck Patterns

Take five to ten minutes to check in about how participants experienced identifying their stuck patterns. Often a participant will ask whether escape behaviors ever actually eliminate painful private experiences in the long term. Sometimes the answer is yes, and if it is, then those experiences are not the ones that keep coming back to bother people. The things most people do to escape what they don't want to feel tend to not work in the long term. They don't permanently delete those experiences.

If someone identifies a strategy that works in the long term, you may need to do a little troubleshooting. Be careful to challenge the participant respectfully and in a way that seems appropriate for the context—but do challenge them! Consider asking for an example. Then say something along the lines of this: "Okay, so you often do X [behavior] when Y [private experience] shows up and Y goes away, but does it permanently go away? What I mean is do you still experience Y?" It is very likely they'll say yes, meaning that the thought, feeling, sensation, or memory hasn't gone away forever.

Yoga Is Noticing Hooks

In this brief exercise, you'll describe to participants how they can pay closer attention to experiences to avoid the stuck patterns they've identified. It's helpful to explain the concept of hooks as *any* experience that drags a person off in a direction they may not have otherwise chosen for themselves; they are simply reacting to whatever shows up. Functional self-disclosure can also be helpful for describing how hooks work. An example of one of your own hooks can serve as a primer during the discussion and yoga practice, helping participants notice their own hooks.

Begin by pointing at the bottom-left quadrant of the life map and saying, "We have a term for our most difficult thoughts, feelings, sensations, and memories, the stuff we struggle with the most. We call them hooks!" Some participants may look puzzled, so we smile and describe what hooks are and how they work:

A hook is any experience that hooks us and pulls us in a direction that we wouldn't have chosen for ourselves. For example, when I'm feeling frustrated with my brother-in-law, I find myself arguing with him and trying to prove him wrong on issues I feel passionately about. In truth, the person I want to be doesn't argue with him. Now, I could say that he's a hook, or the things he says are, but really it's my own frustration that hooks me and causes me to react. As soon as I bite that hook and react, it's almost as if I'm no longer in control of what happens next, the hook is.

Pause and reflect on your own hooks. One that might show up in the context of the MYACT group is "I'm not a good facilitator or yoga teacher." Whatever shows up for you, we encourage you to be playful in your own modeling of this process, remaining defused from your own stuck patterns of behavior.

Victory (Ujjayi) Breath

After asking participants what came up for them in their pairs and explaining how being stuck in patterns of behavior is what we call "being hooked," we transition into the Victory Breath, also known as Ujjayi (oo-ji-ee) Breath. This exercise, and the second session of MYACT in general, builds upon the practices of week one, so be sure to encourage participants to be present with (or mindful of) their experience during this exercise. Because you'll need to briefly describe and demonstrate the Victory Breath, we recommend that you have a strong understanding of the technique yourself.

Rather than simply breathing in and out through the nose, you'll be teaching participants a slow three-part form of breathing. (Pregnant women should not hold their breath and should instead continue breathing normally through this exercise.) Some participants will naturally have success with the Victory Breath based on their biology, the shape of their body, or the size of their nostrils. However, it's a skill that requires practice, and some participants may need extra guidance and explanation. An experienced yoga practitioner will inhale for approximately five seconds, hold the breath for approximately five seconds, and exhale for approximately five seconds.

Describing the Victory (Ujjayi) Breath

We often tell participants that the Victory Breath mimics the ocean sound you might hear when you put a seashell up to your ear. Less poetically, it sounds like Darth Vader. "Fogging the mirror" is one of the methods we employ to teach Ujjayi Breath.

Today we're going to learn a new breathing practice called Victory or Ujjayi Breath, or what I like to fondly call Darth Vader breathing. Begin by finding a comfortable, upright seated position that doesn't require much effort to sit tall. Start by deepening and lengthening the breath. This breath doesn't have be any particular length or depth or duration; simply inhale and exhale through the nose.

Now, place one of your hands, palm facing toward you, about six to eight inches from your mouth. Imagine that the hand in front of you is a mirror. Inhale through the nose, and as you exhale through the mouth pretend that you're fogging up the mirror. Again, inhale through the nose and exhale to fog the mirror. It's okay if you make weird noises; it's part of the process. [*Do a few rounds of this breathing so participants grow more comfortable and familiar with it.*]

Now, instead of inhaling through the nose, inhale through the mouth, but as you inhale breathe in a way that pulls the fog off the mirror. Make sure the inhale is relaxed and easy. If you get too aggressive with the open-mouth inhale, the back of the throat will get really dry, and you'll probably end up coughing. [When we teach this in class, we like to think about and use the imagery of the Dementors from the Harry Potter films, who suck the souls out of people.]

Next, as you exhale through the mouth, halfway through the exhale close your mouth but keep trying to fog the mirror. Inhale through the mouth. Exhale through the mouth, and halfway through the exhale close the mouth. [*Do a few rounds of fogging the mirror with a closed mouth.*]

Now, inhale through the mouth and exhale with the mouth closed fully. Can you now see why I call it Darth Vader breathing?

When this last step feels more comfortable to you and the participants, you can explore keeping the mouth closed on the inhale as well. Slowness is key to the Victory Breath. Remind participants that if they start to feel light-headed, this is not enlightenment. They should consider taking a break and coming back to the Victory Breath later. Also, know that from an ayurvedic perspective, Ujjayi Breath is considered a heating and stimulating breath. As you practice this breath yourself and teach it to participants, be aware that at times, some may become overstimulated. As with functional contextualism, the moment-to-moment experience of what's happening is very important when practicing this breathing pattern.

At the end of this breathing exercise, ask participants to share what thoughts came up for them, and if the difficult thoughts they often struggle with outside of session came up. Then move into the yoga practice for week two. Remember to encourage participants to notice their hooks. The yoga sequence comprises the following poses:

- Table

- Cat and Cow

- Drunken Table

- Child's Pose

- Seated Sun Salutation

- Lying Windshield Wiper

- Seated Forward Fold

The yoga practice in this second session introduces new warm-up postures, transitions into the familiar practice of Seated Sun Salutation, and finishes with new cool-down postures. With an agile group of participants, you may wish to use Standing Half-Sun or Standing Full-Sun Salutations, described in sessions four and seven, respectively.

Table

Come to all fours. Stack the wrists under the shoulders and knees under the hips so that the arms and thighs are perpendicular to the floor.

Allow the spine to find a neutral position. Add a little spread through the fingers. Create a sensation of rooting down from the shoulders, through the arms, and evenly into the palms of the hands and fingers. The rooting down helps to ensure that you're not transmitting all of your weight through the wrists and collapsing them.

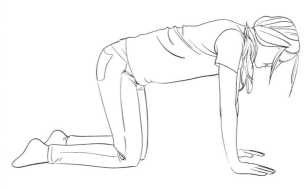

Feel the breath moving in and out, actively but not aggressively. If the wrists or knees are sensitive, you can stack a blanket or towel under one or both of these areas. If the wrists are feeling compressed, there is the option to come up onto the knuckles or fingertips so the wrists are straight. Alternatively, you can also place the forearms on yoga blocks placed at their highest position.

Cat and Cow

Start on the hands and knees with the arms and thighs perpendicular to the floor. If there is some sensitivity in or around the knees or wrists, place a blanket under one or both of these areas. Add a light spread through the fingers and root down from the shoulders, through the arms, and into the hands so that you're not transmitting your weight into the wrists and collapsing them.

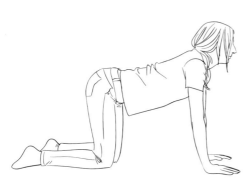
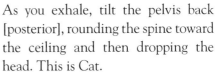

As you notice the natural rhythm of your breath, on an inhale, tilt the pelvis forward [anterior] by lifting the sit bones toward the ceiling, bringing the low belly closer to the floor. Open the chest toward the front of the mat and then lift the head. This is Cow.

As you exhale, tilt the pelvis back [posterior], rounding the spine toward the ceiling and then dropping the head. This is Cat.

Keep the arms straight throughout the movement. Try to start each movement at the pelvis and move up the spine so that the head moves last in the sequence.

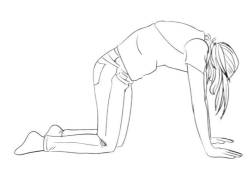

As you're inhaling into Cow, when you get to the upper back, slightly reduce how hard you're pressing from the shoulders into the hands so you feel the shoulder blades move closer to the spine [retraction]. This will help open the chest.

As you exhale into Cat, increase this rooting from the shoulders into the hands so you feel the shoulder blades move slightly away from the spine [protraction], adding some width across the upper back.

We like to suggest that participants imagine the movement as a wave, and the pelvis is the ocean and the head is the shore. Allow the breath to stay long and slow but easy during these Cat and Cow tilts. This will give participants more time to feel the movement happening.

Drunken Table (Bird Dog)

Start this pose in Table.

On an inhale, reach the right arm toward the front of your mat but keep the fingertips on the floor. If it feels appropriate, lift the fingertips off the mat and reach the arm forward, with the palm facing in toward the middle of the mat, like you're going to shake someone's hand. Notice how much more stability is required with the arm raised. Do your best to keep the shoulders level to the floor.

On an exhale, extend the left leg back straight but keep the toes on the floor. Just know that this is an okay place to stay if it feels like enough work. Check in with the breath. Is it smooth or labored? Remember that in this style of yoga, we're using the breath as a barometer for attention and what the nervous system is communicating. [In class we say, "Try not to sacrifice the smoothness of your breath just to get further into a posture."]

Alternatively, keeping the pelvis and low spine neutral, lift the left leg away from the floor. As the leg lifts, do your best to keep the pelvis parallel to the floor. As you hold this position, it's natural for some shaking and adjusting to happen. It's important to not hold your breath, rather allow it to move smoothly. If the breath is getting labored or feels restricted, back off to an easier variation so that the breath can support the posture.

Have participants stay in this position for three to ten breaths. The release is the opposite of the way you went into the pose: lower the foot, bend the knee, return the hand to the floor under the shoulder. Repeat for the opposite side.

Child's Pose

Start this pose in Table.

Bring the legs together. Move the hips back toward the heels, folding the torso over the thighs and bringing the forehead to the floor. The top of the feet should rest on the mat rather than having the toes curled under. If the top of the feet or the shins are tight, try placing a rolled-up towel under the front of the ankles for additional support.

The arms stay toward the front of the mat, or you can bring them back beside the torso so that the fingers point back. The spine will definitely have some roundness in this position. It's okay if the hips don't touch the heels. That's not the goal of Child's Pose.

If you notice sensitivity around the knees or tightness in the fronts of the thighs [quadriceps], you can place a block or two between the shins and under the hips. This will allow the hips to settle onto something and decrease the pressure in the knees. Other options for this pose include taking the knees wider while you keep the toes together. This variation allows the torso to settle in between the legs and the spine to find more length rather than roundness. There is still the option to rest the hips on a block or two.

If you start to feel tension around the upper back, shoulders, or neck with the knees wide and arms forward, it's a good idea to place a prop under the chest so the upper spine doesn't collapse.

As you hold this pose for three to ten (maybe even twenty) breaths, keep encouraging participants to notice what kinds of sensations arise, and what kind of thinking shows up, if any. If participants' mobility is limited, Child's Pose can bring up intense sensations. In class we might say, "Be aware of the tendency to try and convince yourself that you can make this comfortable when you're uncomfortable or even in pain. If Child's Pose and your body are not getting along, your job is not to make them get along." If this position is too uncomfortable for some participants, they can roll onto their back and hug their knees in to their chest.

Once you are finished with Child's Pose, complete **Seated Sun Salutation**, as outlined in session one.

Lying Windshield Wiper

Lie on your back, with your feet flat on the floor. Have the feet separated a comfortable distance. Take your arms out your sides, with your arms and hands in line with the shoulders, and the palms facing up toward the ceiling.

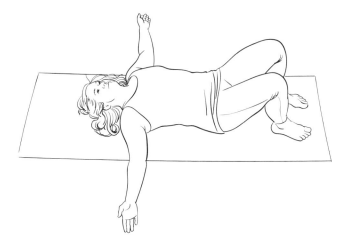

If it's uncomfortable to have the arms in this position, it's okay to move them closer to the torso. As you tune in to the movement of your breath, on a slow exhale, allow the knees to drop toward the right side of your mat as your head turns to the left, coming into a small twist.

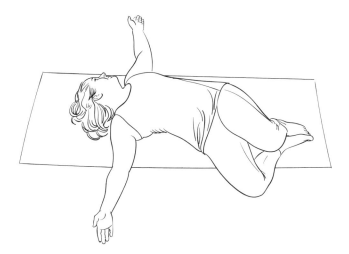

As you inhale, bring the legs and the head back to center. On an exhale, allow the legs to drop toward the left side of your mat as the head turns to the right. Inhale as you return to center.

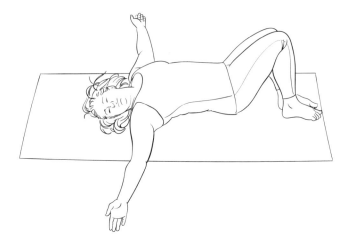

With the rhythm of the breath, continue moving the legs from side to side, like a windshield wiper, always moving the head in the opposite direction of the legs. If your body starts to give you negative feedback, try slowing the movement. Sometimes, if we move too quickly, the body will start to seize up as a way to stop us from moving. This is known as protective tension. We want the body to have enough time to adapt to the movement, which is why slowness is such an important concept in the practice of yoga.

If slowing the movement down doesn't help, decrease how far you're allowing the legs to drop toward the floor. Listen to your body, because it provides you with the most important feedback about how well you're moving. As you continue to move, notice any thoughts that might arise around how far you can move or how far you wish you could move or how far your mind tells you that you ought to be able to move. To stay present in the movement, keep practicing syncing the movement and the breathing.

For a more advanced version, participants can have their feet lifted away from the floor and their knees more toward the chest. This variation definitely requires more stability, but it might be available for some participants. It's important to keep reinforcing that the practice is not necessarily about doing hard physical work or getting to the next level as quickly as we can. We encourage participants to work with what's present and what's available.

After completing Lying Windshield Wiper, it's time to have participants cool down. Do **Seated Forward Fold**, as described in session one.

Group Dialogue: Debriefing Yoga Practice

Encourage participants to sit at the front of their yoga mats in a seated posture that is comfortable: "Moving in your own time, find yourself seated at the front of your mat." Transition into debriefing the practice by asking, "What did you notice in that practice? Did you get hooked?" Spend a few minutes debriefing the practice and talking about what hooks participants noticed.

Know Your Hooks

Now that the concept of hooks has been explained, and participants have been guided through a brief yoga practice with a debrief encouraging them to share any hooks they noticed, the following exercise brings their attention to their hooks and behavior that might show up outside of session. This more formal defusion exercise uses a brief facilitator introduction and a worksheet (Gordon & Borushok, 2017) for more small-group work, challenging participants to reflect on their problematic behaviors and the potential antecedent events that may have hooked them, triggering the behaviors. You can download the worksheet, along with other accessories for this book, at http://www.newharbinger.com/42358. Consider using the following script, which is about getting to know one's hooks.

So now that we've had the chance to look at how we get stuck trying to escape, avoid, or control our most painful experiences, let's pause for a moment and ask ourselves what we'd like to be about, if we weren't working so hard to not feel what we don't want to feel. We like to call the things that get in the way of living a meaningful life, the things that impact our behavior in a problematic way, hooks. A hook is something that entices you to bite it, and once you're hooked, you react without thinking.

Can I use a simple example with all of you?

Imagine we're all fish swimming out in the ocean, and we come across a shiny hook dangling in the water. Now, I don't know what a hook is, but you do. You see me start swimming toward the hook, getting ready to bite it. What do you do? Remember, we're fish. [Participants often suggest bumping you out of the way, slapping you with a fin, getting you to go somewhere else.]

Exactly! You maybe bump me out of the way and say, "Hey, don't eat that! If you're looking for some good food I can show you a place with excellent kelp." And we would all swim off together.

Would we go up close and examine the hook, knock off some flecks of metal and try to figure out what it's made of? Would we follow the line all the way up to see who placed the hook there, such as our parents, or a bully from school, or a stranger? Would we put up signs and call for "Hook Awareness Month"? No! We're fish. We'd swim away and not give the hook another thought.

Know Your Hooks

A hook is any experience that impacts your behavior. It can be direct, like stubbing your toe and reacting in anger, or indirect, like seeing a social media post that reminds you of an old friend who hurt you, which causes you to spend time thinking about painful memories and canceling plans with your current friends.

1. What happened? Write down a situation in which you did something problematic. What did you do?

_____

_____

_____

2. Pay attention. Write down what private experiences, such as thoughts, feelings, sensations, or memories, showed up for you and triggered the problematic behavior.

_____

_____

_____

3. Is the experience a hook? Here's how you can tell: Did the painful experience impact your behavior in a problematic way? If so, write down the name of that hook (for example, "My sadness hook," "My I'm unlovable hook," and so on).

_____

_____

_____

4. Prepare. What would the person you want to be do when your hook shows up? Bite it and react? Engage in the same behavior? If not, write down what you would choose to do differently when the hook shows up.

_____

_____

_____

5. Go out and notice your hooks. Noticing your hooks is a life skill. You don't get to choose whether you have hooks or not, but you can choose how you respond to them and how you interact with them.

But, for better or worse we are humans, and that means that hooks can show up as physical things, such as a certain place or person, or as content our minds make up. We can be walking outside on a nice sunny day and, BAM! All of a sudden a hook shows up in our mind! And if we bite that hook, if we believe it to be true or adhere to its rigid rules or start trying to find ways to get rid of it, we can get so caught up in the hook that it derails our plan for moving toward the who and what that matter to us.

Now, we don't get to choose whether we have hooks or not. Everyone has hooks. But we do get to choose what to do when they show up, if we're paying attention.

Slowing down and noticing what's happening in any given situation is one method for identifying hooks. If you could all take out your Know Your Hooks worksheet I can show you what I mean.

Now, call to mind a recent situation when you behaved in a way you deemed problematic. It might be a time that, after you had a moment to breathe, you wish you'd handled something differently. And if you could get a do-over, you would handle it differently. Write down exactly what happened under number 1.

As you're thinking about that situation and writing it down, consider what was going on inside of you at the time. Did a thought or a memory pop into your head? Did you notice unpleasant physical sensations? Did you experience a painful emotion? Write down whatever you noticed happening inside you under number 2.

Is what you put down under number 2 a hook? Did it influence your behavior in some way? If so, write down that hook under number 3. You can give it a name, such as "My anger hook," or "I'm a terrible parent hook," or "I'm exhausted hook." Whatever showed up, give it a name.

Now, if you could go back in time, back into yourself right before engaging in the behavior you wish you hadn't, what would you choose to do instead when that hook showed up? What would the person you want to be do in that situation? Write it down under number 4.

And finally, take a moment to pause and notice that you're seeing your hooks and choosing to do something different when they show up. Consider what it means to see your hooks before they influence you, before you bite them. Can you see how noticing creates choice?

End the exercise by instructing participants to notice their hooks and to pay attention to them on purpose. The goal is to impact their behavior. We want to encourage them to approach with curiosity the difficult experiences that typically shut them down—that have them trying to escape, avoid, or control. Rather than being pushed around by their experiences and goaded into reacting, we want them to feel in control of and to be intentional about what they do next.

Group Dialogue: Debriefing Know Your Hooks

After everyone has completed the Know Your Hooks worksheet, take a few minutes to debrief, asking participants what they noticed during the exercise. You may want to note that even though people named different hooks, everyone has hooks. If multiple people have similar hooks, you can point this out to normalize the experience.

Session Two Home Practice: Movement, Intention, and Goal Setting

Transition into the home practice by linking the concept of patterned living (samskāra) with noticing hooks. We choose to not use the language of "letting go" of or "not biting" hooks when introducing the home practice. Instead, we focus on the inevitability of hooks and encourage participants to engage with noticing: "You're going to leave this session today and get hooked. It just happens. Hooks can show up anywhere, and when they do, we tend to go back to old patterns. For our home practice, we're going to set goals and notice the hooks that show up."

The Purposeful STEPS worksheet (available for download at http://www.newharbinger .com/42358) will help guide participants through identifying a values-based goal to work toward. After completing the worksheet, each participant will fill out an index card. One side of the index card is for SMART goals. You'll ask participants to translate what they wrote in the Purposeful STEPS worksheet using the SMART acronym. On the other side, they'll write out an implementation intention for their stated goal, as well as identify different behavioral cues to remind them of their goal. We incorporate the implementation intention to increase the likelihood that a new behavior will become an established pattern of life, and also as a way to demonstrate that rules aren't bad. Rather, our focus is that some behaviors can bring us closer to the life we want, whereas others won't. We want to encourage a flexible and functional way of viewing behaviors, and we do this by providing a lot of different examples of how to introduce, practice, and use this philosophy of functional contextualism.

The session two home practice focuses on the concept of movement and includes goals related to health, exercise, and movement. Given that participants decided to address their mental health through a group therapy that includes the active practice of yoga, it's probably safe to assume that they have a value related to being more active or increasing movement in everyday life. Plus, as yoga is a movement practice, practicing skills related to these goals may be an easy transition for participants because they'll seem familiar. Some participants may choose to practice certain yoga poses or sequences at home. Here's a script that we like to use.

The work that we do here, in this room, is only a small part of the work you will be doing over the coming weeks. After all, we only see you for a small portion of your week. If this is the only time that you focus on the changes you'd like to make in your life and to practice the skills we're developing, then your progress will be much slower. That's why every week, we have an at-home practice that focuses on some aspect of your life and provides you the opportunity to bring to life in a concrete, actionable way some of the abstract principles we're teaching through MYACT. Today we're going to touch briefly on the many ways we set intentions and the strategies for ensuring we successfully take steps toward the life we want to create for ourselves. We're going to do this through a conversation about movement.

Because you chose to come to a group therapy that incorporates yoga, I'm going to assume that movement, exercise, and physical activity are important to you for some reason. What are some of the values you have around physical activity, exercise, or simply moving more? What led you to choose this yoga-based group rather than, say, a traditional therapy group or a tai chi class? [Generally, participants will respond with specific reasons why they picked yoga.]

Great! There's some interesting research about physical activity going around. We all know that exercise is important for our health and helps us in many ways, but what you may not know is that new research has debunked the rule that we need only get 150 minutes of exercise per week. Many experts used to believe that if you exercised 150 minutes per week (30 minutes of walking 5 times per week), that it didn't matter if you were sedentary the rest of the time (while commuting, sitting at work, or engaging in leisure activities, such as watching Netflix). Now we know that exercise and movement are two different things, and that they impact our health in different ways. What does this mean for us? If we exercise for that minimum of 150 minutes per week but remain sedentary the rest of the time, we are still at an increased risk for a lot of serious health problems. One of our goals in this group is to work toward a whole health approach to living. We want to make sure that we're taking the best care of ourselves in values-consistent ways so that we can do the things that matter to us and live a long, fulfilling life. One of the ways we achieve these goals is to create a life of movement, finding ways to engage in the world that increase our steps in the right direction and keep us healthy.

When we talk about how we want to live our lives, we're talking about much more than goals: we are talking about who and what are most meaningful to us and what a fulfilling life looks like for us. As we've already discussed, we cannot move toward who and what matter to us without knowing what they are. The same is true about moving toward what's important to us. It's a struggle when we don't know what steps to take and when hooks get in our way and pull us in the wrong direction (for example, watching television because you're tired after work even though you planned to walk with your partner after dinner). Everyone here seems to have at least one value tied to movement or activity, so today we're going to use those values to create workable goals that will, literally and figuratively, help us take steps to increase movement in our daily life. We'll also discuss common barriers that may show up along the way.

Using the Purposeful STEPS worksheet, and keeping in mind the conversations we've had about our life maps, identify one value related to movement. It can be a who or what that you put in the bottom-right quadrant of your life map, or it can even be a quality or characteristic you want to embody. Then answer the questions to set a goal for moving toward that value, either on your own or with others. It can be as simple as taking a walk outside after dinner, completing physical therapy exercises at home, doing squats during commercial breaks, parking farther from the store you're going to, or going out dancing with friends or a partner.

Notice that the last part of the worksheet talks about setbacks. While there may be physical barriers to achieving your goal, we've also learned today how hooks can set us on a different path than the one we'd like to choose. Be sure to identify a couple of hooks that may show up as you work toward this goal.

Next, using the worksheet as a guide, fill out an index card. On one side, write out your goal using the acronym SMART.

S stands for "specific." Just as you did on the worksheet, write out the specific movement goal you created for yourself.

M stands for "measurable." Write down how you will measure your progress toward this goal. How will you know you completed the goal? For example, you could write it down in a planner and cross it off when you've completed it, or you could use a phone app to track your progress.

A stands for "attainable." Sometimes we have a goal but not all the resources to actually achieve the goal. What resources do you need to complete this goal? You may need to ask others to support you with this goal or to help you with it, or maybe you need to buy certain materials to complete your goal or learn a specific skill.

R stands for "relevant." Why is this goal important? Write out a sentence that captures your value.

T stands for "time bound." When will this goal be completed by? If it is a recurring goal, which days and times will you regularly complete it? Be specific. Be sure to choose something you can complete before our next session.

Excellent! Now please turn the index card over. We're going to briefly identify some simple strategies for increasing your odds of taking that first step toward what matters to you.

First, we're going to create something called an implementation intention, which is quite simple. It's a statement or rule for yourself that you will *do* something when you *encounter* something. An implementation intention follows this general format: if situation X is encountered, then I will perform behavior Y.

When forming an implementation intention, it's important to link a future situational cue (for example, brushing my teeth) with a goal-directed response (for example, practice five minutes of mindful breathing). For example, "If *I brush my teeth*, then I will *practice five minutes of mindful breathing.*"

And finally, we will write down a few behavioral cues. A behavioral cue is something we use to remind us to work toward a goal. A behavioral cue for the example of practicing five minutes of mindful breathing while brushing one's teeth could be putting a sticky note that says "five minutes, mindful breathing" on the bathroom mirror. You could also set an alarm on your phone to remind you of this goal around the time you generally brush your teeth, or set a timer next to your toothbrush. It doesn't matter what the cue is as long as it helps remind you to follow through with your goal.

Above all, remember to be kind to yourself as you move forward. If you don't complete your goal this week, that's okay. Make sure you take time to identify what hooks got in your way. It may be that your first step in this process is noticing the hooks before attempting to alter the behavior.

Which implementation intention and behavioral cues can you come up with for your stated goal? Write them on the back of the index card.

Would anyone be willing to share their value and goal?

Purposeful STEPS

Living a values-driven life involves getting out of your head and stepping into the world. What will your next step be?

My value is: _____

1. Specific

   - Write down a goal related to your stated value. Remember, this should be a behavior you want to begin doing. Describe it as specifically and as detailed as possible.

     _____

     _____

     _____

     _____

   - What steps will you take to help you reach your goal?

     _____

     _____

     _____

     _____

     _____

2. Tracking

   - How will you track this goal?

     _____

     _____

     _____

     _____

     _____

     _____

3. End date

- Set an end date for your goal. If you meet the goal by the end date, determine what your next goal is.

- If you didn't meet the end date, examine your STEPS to see which modifications need to be made. If you felt stuck, fill out a life map. And REPEAT!

    I will reach my goal by: _____

4. Possible

- Is this goal possible?

- Do you have all of the skills and resources you need to complete this goal? If not, how can you get them? Who can help?

    _____

    _____

    _____

    _____

    _____

5. Setbacks

- Which barriers, both private and observable, could potentially arise that would get in the way of you reaching your goal?

- What can you do to prevent setbacks?

    _____

    _____

    _____

    _____

    _____

    _____

    _____

Ending Savasana: What Matters Is What Hurts

Invite participants to lie down in a circle (if possible), with their head at the top of their mat, feet pointed away from the group. Turn the lights down, if possible, but not off completely. Invite participants to relax their eyelids. They can close their eyes or leave them open.

As we're coming to the end of this practice, take a breath on purpose, pause, and notice how you're feeling in this moment. Whatever shows up, acknowledge it and breathe it in, welcoming your whole experience here in this room.

Challenge yourself to inhale and scan your body. Notice any tension you may be holding, such as a tight jaw with clenched teeth. On an exhale, breathe all the way out and allow your body to soften, feeling the tension loosen. Take a few breaths in your own time on purpose, breathing in to notice and exhaling to soften.

During this session, we discussed our most difficult experiences and how they impact our behavior.

Reflect on a difficult thought, feeling, sensation, or memory that hooks you. Really come in contact with it, identifying the situations in which it shows up in your life.

Whatever comes to mind, breathe it in, pause, and breathe out to be here, witnessing your struggles.

Even this very act of paying attention to the difficult moments in your life that cause you to get stuck creates awareness, and with that awareness, you can practice slowing into this moment, holding your difficult moments lightly, and with that slowing, you give yourself space to choose what you do next.

In the space that you now have between your thoughts, feelings, sensations, and memories, begin to bring motion into your body, wiggling the fingers, slowly rotating the wrists. Notice your reactions as you wake the body up.

In your own time, roll onto your side, using your hand to push yourself up. Come to be seated at the front of your mat to begin our good-bye ritual.

Once all participants are seated at the top of their mat, end this second session of MYACT as you ended session one, with chanting, sharing appreciations, and a closing posture.

Working with Individuals

- Complete the functional analysis of the client's life map as a discussion. You may still choose to write down responses on a whiteboard or piece of paper.

- Rather than using the Know Your Hooks worksheet, you may choose to have a conversation about hooks and then send the client home with the worksheet to practice identifying hooks based on their experiences during the week.

- Depending on your client's therapy goals, you may alter the goal they identify as part of the Purposeful STEPS worksheet, and either complete the worksheet in session or give it to them for homework.

- You can shorten the yoga practice by reducing the number of poses while still maintaining a focus on noticing hooks.

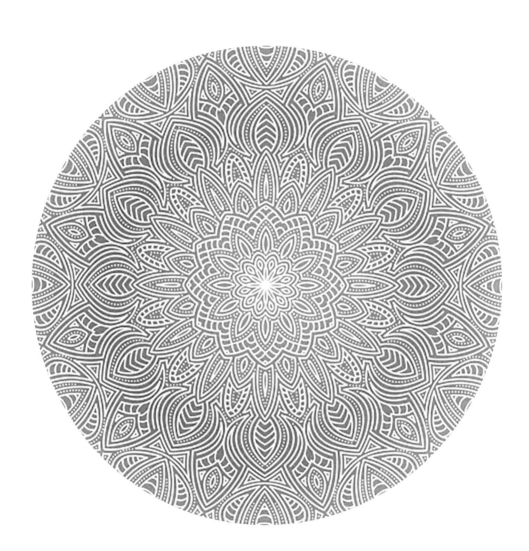

Dhyāna

In the third session of MYACT, we invite participants to once more focus their attention on the present moment and acknowledge attempts to escape, avoid, or control painful experiences. We revisit the concept that attempting to control our pain doesn't work and often leads to suffering, often called creative hopelessness in ACT, by identifying common avoidance strategies and then helping participants refocus their attention from pain to what is important. Our goal is to make a sufficient intellectual and experiential argument, across multiple occasions, that acceptance is a process we continually work on. Dhyāna, this week's theme, complements and reflects the importance of acceptance. *Dhyāna* means an openness to experience through inquiring, reflecting, and understanding. Sessions one and two put participants in contact with their pain, and this third session demonstrates that new growth and living can be done in spite of it through acceptance and dhyāna.

As facilitators, we often pause when a participant describes a painful situation, listen intently, and then inquire why that particular hurt matters—why it's important. More often than not, participants can identify someone or something directly connected to their pain. This third session encourages acceptance in the service of growth, or deeper connection with values.

Beginning Meditation: Paying Attention

You may need to remind participants to start the session in silence with Savasana or any posture, including sitting on a chair, that is appropriate for them. This beginning meditation will be a familiar present-moment-focused exercise for participants, but its scope expands to include novel perspective taking. By this third session, participants should be starting to show a higher level of comfort with the beginning meditation.

Taking stock of whatever you're bringing into this room with you, take an extralong inhale. Noticing what occurs to you here, now: sensations, thoughts, feelings, memories, judgments, comparisons. Whatever shows up for you, exhale, feeling the sensations of breath in your body.

Remember coming here today. Really picture yourself before you arrived. What were you doing? Be there behind your eyes and breathe this memory in. Remember yourself walking, driving, or however you commuted to this space. What is it like to be there behind your eyes? Pause and really feel what shows up for you.

Feeling the sensations of being in this room, noticing sounds, the sound of my voice. Noticing the sensations of your body being supported. Bring your awareness to the sensations of breathing. When you're ready, bringing some motion into the body, whether it's a wiggle of the fingers, a rotation of the wrists, a motion in the neck as you turn the head from side to side. Allow your body to awaken.

Coming back to this room, opening your eyes. If you're supine in Savasana or another relaxation pose, rolling to your right and using your left arm to raise yourself, coming to a seated position.

Look around for a moment. Notice the faces of the other participants in this room. Let's all take an inhale on purpose together. Exhale. Breathe all the way out as we return to our work together.

Group Dialogue: Debriefing Beginning Meditation

Take a breath, and in silence, look at each of the participants, perhaps making eye contact, smiling, nodding, or otherwise acknowledging each participant. Do a visual check-in. Break the silence by asking, "What did you notice in that meditation?" Take a few minutes to debrief their responses.

Group Dialogue: Debriefing Home Practice

Take ten minutes to check in with participants about their experience of the last session's home practice. The point of the debrief is to explore with participants what they noticed, regardless of whether they "achieved" their goals or not. Here are a couple of helpful questions to ask:

Before we move on, how did everyone feel after they went home last week?

Did you have any difficulty or success with implementing your movement goal?

How was it to do this practice?

What did you notice while doing it?

Did any hooks show up? If so, what did you do when you noticed a hook?

Escape, Avoidance, and Control Checklist

After the group debrief, have participants break into groups of two. Encourage them to pick a new partner. Hand out the Escape, Avoidance, and Control Checklist, instructing participants to interview each other. They should check off thinking and doing strategies first and then describe their own strategies not included in the checklist. To finish, each participant should review their strategies and note what they have cost them—that is, the toll they've paid for attempting to escape, avoid, and control. You can download the worksheet, along with other accessories for this book, at http://www.newharbinger.com/42358.

Group Dialogue: Debriefing the Escape, Avoidance, and Control Checklist

Invite participants to rejoin the group, and then debrief their experience of completing the checklist by asking what they noticed. Some participants may still take for granted their level of sensitivity to content that shows up for them during the small-group exercises, and they may make comments such as "I already know all the avoidance strategies I use," or "I didn't notice anything new." We try to point this out in a reinforcing and playful way: "Isn't this the kind of stuff we notice but don't pay attention to explicitly, really keeping track of how our avoidance strategies impact us?"

Once more, we'd like to encourage you, as the facilitator of a MYACT group, to functionally self-disclose, modeling the position of mutual vulnerability. Specifically, discuss how expending more effort to fight against pain and trying to improve escape, avoidance, and control strategies doesn't necessarily lead to better outcomes. You may want to link this conversation to the functional analysis of the previous session: "Remember last week when we walked through a painful situation using the life map and identified an avoidance loop that many of us get stuck in? Sometimes, our efforts to escape or avoid pain feels productive, but after a while, it's like we're just running in circles and end up exhausted and in worse shape than when we started. They don't help us move forward." This debrief leads perfectly into discussing the theme of the session: dhyāna, being open to pain so as to better understand the impact of rejecting pain.

Escape, Avoidance, and Control Checklist

Check off the strategies you have tried to use to escape, avoid, or control your painful thoughts, feelings, sensations, and memories.

Thinking

- ☐ Worrying
- ☐ Dwelling on the past
- ☐ Questioning yourself
- ☐ Blaming yourself
- ☐ Blaming others
- ☐ Blaming the world
- ☐ Thinking "It's not fair"
- ☐ Thinking "If only…"
- ☐ Fantasizing about suicide
- ☐ Fantasizing about killing someone else
- ☐ Suppressing or pushing away thoughts
- ☐ Imagining escaping your job, school, or family
- ☐ Analyzing yourself

Doing

- ☐ Isolating
- ☐ Eating
- ☐ Self-harming
- ☐ Arguing or complaining
- ☐ Drinking alcohol or caffeine
- ☐ Using drugs recreationally
- ☐ Misusing prescription drugs
- ☐ Physically acting out or fighting
- ☐ Hooking up or being sexually promiscuous
- ☐ Shopping or spending money
- ☐ Bingeing on movies, TV shows, or video games
- ☐ Saying no to opportunities

Write Your Own

Write down strategies not listed on this worksheet that you've tried.

_____

_____

_____

_____

_____

Yoga Is Self-Acceptance

Session three provides participants a more advanced yoga practice. These physically challenging postures offer participants an excellent opportunity to practice self-acceptance. For example, some participants may notice the impulse to push harder, striving for specific outcomes, such as doing a pose even if that means sacrificing form or straining the body. Others may become stuck on thoughts about their inability to do a difficult pose and feel the urge to opt out of persisting, or perhaps they'll attempt a strenuous posture without first checking in with what the body can handle. Encourage participants to notice their urges to push harder or retreat and to practice a willingness to feel the urge instead of engaging in it. They can also choose an alternative behavior, such as taking on a relaxation posture to catch their breath or holding a challenging posture for one or two more breaths.

Before beginning the yoga practice, facilitate a brief discussion about practicing self-acceptance through yoga. In ACT, there is an important distinction made between acceptance and resignation. The implication of "resignation" is that things will always be the way they are, unless by some twist of fate they miraculously change by themselves. Participants may think that you want them to "suck it up" or "just deal with it" when you use the word "acceptance" while practicing yoga. It's important to clarify that real acceptance, in this moment, is more of a "this is the ways things are right now" kind of attitude. In yoga, we say that every moment is fresh and new, which is not a lie. Everything *is* changing all the time. Earlier we said that yoga is always inviting us to truly be ourselves, and one of the hardest things in practice or in life is to meet this body and this mind as they are in this moment, and into the next moment, without sticking to the idea of the old you.

Steve loves to play baseball. Prior to and during baseball season, he trains to make sure that he plays well and avoids injury. Because he's doing things with his body that he doesn't do during the off-season, his body feels and is very different. Because of this "new body," Steve has to revamp how he moves through his yoga practice. His practice during baseball season is much different than that during the off-season.

Yoga tells us that our ability to feel sensations and breathing is our most direct way of working with present-moment awareness. It is through our ability and willingness to consciously slow down and connect to our immediate experience that we can get direct insight into how we tend to meet each moment. If this is truly the way that it is right now, how can we meet the moment as it arises? By allowing for some room to witness where and how we are, how we're relating to where and how, and the possible options we have ahead of us.

You'll now conduct the third yoga sequence, comprising the following poses:

- Cat and Cow

- Seated Sun Salutation

- Mountain

- Warrior 1

- Warrior 2

- Side Angle

- Triangle

- Bridge

- Legs Up the Wall

Begin with a brief warm-up to connect the body with the practice. Start with **Cat and Cow** (described in session two) and **Seated Sun Salutation** (described in session one).

After warming up, you'll move on to what are known as foundational poses. They are "foundational" inasmuch as they are popular contemporary poses frequently associated with and used in contemporary postural yoga. The poses we use in the MYACT protocol are common and likely form the foundation of the yoga classes you or your participants have attended. They literally help build a foundation because they are strengthening and stability poses.

Mountain

Stand at the front of your mat, with the feet hip-width apart. We'll start with what I like to call "floppy mountain," which means that at first, you're not really trying to pose yourself or stand up tall. If you notice a tendency to hyperextend the knees, sometimes referred to as "locking out," add a small bend to your stance. With a relaxed body, allow your weight to settle down into the feet.

From "floppy mountain," begin to root down from your hips, through the legs, and evenly into the soles of the feet. Ideally when you root down just enough, you'll feel a slight rising sensation through the spine. This rise is not something you force, rather it's a by-product of or response to the rooting down. If you push down too much, you'll feel the upper body pulled down toward the feet. This is not what we're looking for. ["Root down to rise up" is a common statement in yoga classes.]

Take some time to play around with this sensation on your mat. Root down just a little bit at a time and feel the response you get. Notice the sensations as the rest of the body responds, how the breath might get stifled if you're holding yourself too rigidly.

Once you're rooted through the legs, start to lightly draw the shoulder blades in toward the spine. This will help to broaden the chest and collarbones. Make sure that your spine doesn't move into a backbend (spinal extension) as you draw the shoulder blades in.

As you maintain the rooting through the legs, along with the shoulder blades pulled in, lightly reach up through the top of the head to lengthen the back of the neck without tilting the chin up or down. Be aware that reaching up with too much effort will deweight the feet. So reach up only as much as you can while remaining grounded.

As you establish Mountain, feel the breath moving fluidly throughout the body. Also notice that as you stand up tall and root down that the body will still waver slightly. This is okay. The posture is meant to help the body find a tall and stable position while allowing it to explore its own inherent stability. As Sōtō Zen founder Eihei Dōgen would say, "Even mountains are walking."

Warrior 1

Stand at the front of your mat, with feet hip-width apart. Keeping the hips square with the front of the mat [Placing your hands on the hips to make sure they stay square is a useful aid for proprioception.] and the spine neutral, step the right leg back approximately two to three feet to find a lunge. Pivoting on the ball of the right foot, externally rotate the right thigh outward to bring the right heel to the floor.

If the pelvis begins to twist away from the front of the mat while bringing the back foot flat, try widening the stance by moving the right foot toward the right side of the mat. If that doesn't allow the hips to square themselves with the front of the mat, try shortening the stance by bringing the right foot toward the front of the mat. Also, if, as you find the lunge, you notice that the spine has moved into a slight backbend, shorten the distance between the feet.

[At this point, we might ask participants to notice any thoughts arising, such as any about how long their stance is. If some of the participants have practiced yoga elsewhere, they may have vastly different ideas about how to approach this lunge, such as forcing the body into a "true" representation of the pose, with a longer stance, rather than the pose that best fits where their body is in the moment. This is one of the reasons why we emphasize approaching asana from the perspectives of functional movement and acceptance.]

Next, add a bend to the left knee, making sure to not move the knee in front of the left ankle. Maintaining a neutral spine, take the arms upward with palms facing one another. Maintain some softness in the shoulders. If the shoulders or neck feel uncomfortable, explore taking the arms wider, lowering them in front of the body more, or bringing the hands to heart center or even back to the hips. If there is any discomfort in the right hip, knee, ankle, or foot, widening or shortening the stance may be very helpful.

Hold this pose for five to ten breaths.

To finish, bring the hands to heart center and step the back foot forward to find Mountain. Take a moment to feel the breath and the response that you're getting from the body before switching to the opposite side. Notice if Mountain feels different having done Warrior 1 on one side and not the other. As you switch sides, the opposite side of the body will feel and function a little differently. Treat this side as *this side*. Use whatever modifications you need to use.

[*Repeat the above sequence for the other side of the body.*]

Warrior 2

Start with a wide-legged stance, facing the side of your mat. Have the feet parallel. The pelvis and spine determine the width of your stance. You want them to be neutral, so widen your stance accordingly.

You may need to slow down while widening your stance in order to feel the point at which the spine begins to enter into a backbend and the pelvis tips forward. Again, a neutral stance is important.

Externally rotate the right leg so that the right foot faces the front of the mat, and internally rotate the left leg slightly so that the foot angles in five to ten degrees. The feet will be in a relative heel-to-arch alignment, with the front heel lining up with the back arch.

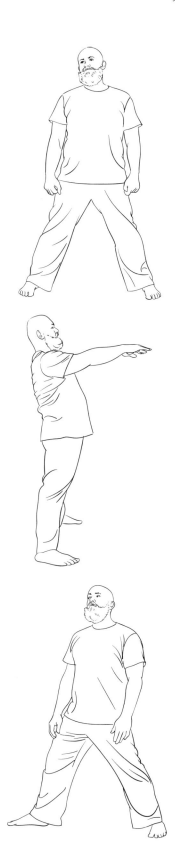

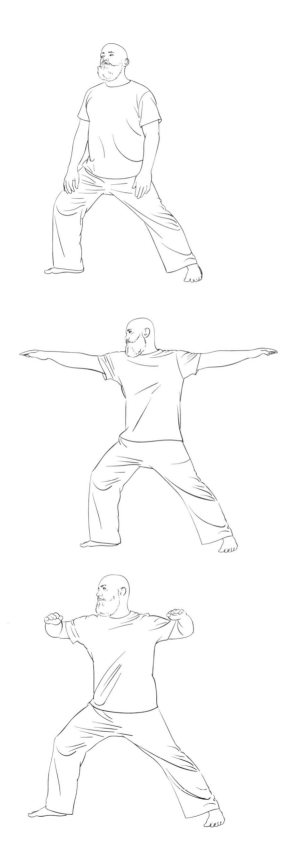

Bend the right knee. Ideally, it sits directly above the ankle, but it shouldn't be in front of it. If this position stresses the knee, reduce the bend. There is no need to have the leg bent that much. Having the knee directly over the ankle might be a position to work up to.

Lift the arms out to the sides parallel to the floor, with the palms facing down.

If the shoulders or neck start to feel overly tight or irritated, keep the upper arms parallel to the floor but bend the elbows so the fingertips face the same direction as the chest and pelvis. This helps decrease the load on the shoulders.

Rotate the neck to the right as much as feels comfortable. Stay here for five to ten breaths. [Cuing students to notice how their breath responds as the body fatigues helps them hold their attention rather than allowing it to stray.] If the breath can't remain smooth and relatively easy in this position, try shortening the stance to the point that the breath can help support the posture and the nervous system can stay relatively calm. [It's common for participants to be resistant to shortening the stance, especially if they already have a yoga practice in which they're used to focusing on longer stances and heavily manipulating the breath. Remind participants about the aims and objectives of this particular style of yoga, and encourage them to follow the guidelines to the best of their ability.]

To finish, lower the arms, bring the head back to center, and align the feet to parallel each other. Just as with Warrior 1, before we do the pose with the other side, you might take some time connecting to the breath, noticing the response from the body, and being aware of any thoughts or feelings arising. As you repeat on the other side, again, remember that this is *this side*, and make any necessary modifications.

Side Angle

Start in the Warrior 2 leg position, right leg forward first, with a bent right knee. Have the hands in the hip creases, like a lobster claw, to feel the sensation of pelvic movement. Doing your best to keep the spine neutral, begin to tilt the pelvis toward the right leg such that your body starts leaning in the direction of the right leg. You're looking for the pelvis to laterally tilt on the thigh bones and not the spine to bend at the waist, creating a C curve. [This is a common mistake people will make to compensate for decreased range of motion in the hips. Be sure to emphasize that to ensure proper form throughout the movement, it's important for the spine to stay neutral.]

Once the pelvis has reached its full range of tilt, bring the right forearm or hand to whatever is available for support, such as your thigh, a block, or a chair. Take the left arm straight out from the shoulder or, if it feels available, sweep it up beside the head, with fingers pointing toward the front of the mat and the palm of the hand facing the floor. This is Side Angle.

It's important that you don't feel as though your arm is doing the job of holding you up. You want to make sure that the hips, legs, and core are doing that job, and that the arm is only there to support that work. Hold for three to ten breaths.

When the time comes to move out of the pose, as you bring the pelvis back level to the floor, try to make sure that the pelvis moves on the thigh bones, and it's not the spine pulling you into a side bend. [This position can also be done with the back against a wall, if balance is an issue.]

Repeat on the other side. As a warm-up, you might have participants keep their hands on their hips and practice tilting the pelvis and then leveling it off five to ten times before you have them hold the position. As always, go with what you're feeling in the session based on the fitness of participants.

Triangle

Start in the Warrior 2 leg position, right leg forward first, but, unlike Side Angle, keep the legs straight, not bent. Be careful not to hyperextend the knees.

Doing your best to keep the spine neutral, begin to tilt the pelvis toward the right leg. Just as in Side Angle, you're looking for the pelvis to laterally tilt on the thigh bones and not the spine bending at the waist. Once the pelvis has reached its full range of tilt, bring the right hand to whatever is available for support, such as your thigh, your shin, a block, or blocks. Take the left arm straight out from the shoulder, pointed up toward the ceiling. If the shoulder, neck, or arm feels irritated in this upward position, it's okay to just rest the hand on the waist.

When the time comes to move out of the pose, try to make sure the movement happens through the pelvis and not the spine as you bring the pelvis back to a level position.

Repeat on the other side. With Triangle, it isn't uncommon for people to place strong meaning or emphasis on going deeper, trying to get a deep stretch by getting the hand closer to the floor. Getting the hand closer to the floor or a block might happen someday for some participants, but it isn't what we're emphasizing in MYACT. Our goal is to be mindful of *how* we move into postures, *how* we hold them, and *how* we move out of them. It's good to remind participants of this.

Bridge

Start lying on your back with your feet flat on the floor. Have the feet separated hip width with the heels approximately ten inches from the hips. [It's common to hear a yoga teacher say, "You'll know when the heels are in the right place when you can tickle them." However, a lot of people tend to add a little side bend in the spine or extend their upper arm bones slightly out of the shoulder sockets to get the tickle. This can lead to pain and improper form, so instead we like to say, "Without moving too much through the pelvis or the spine, walk the heels toward the hips. The goal isn't to get the heels as close to the hips as you can, or to be able to tickle the heels." We usually throw in a joke about having short arms like a T-rex and never being able to tickle our heels.]

Once the legs are in a comfortable position, with the upper arms beside the ribs resting on the floor, bend the elbows ninety degrees so the palms face each other and the fingertips face the ceiling. [We like to call this position "Mr. Roboto arms."]

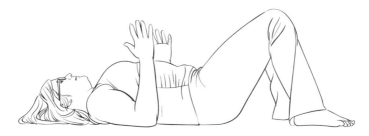

Actively, but not aggressively, begin to root the upper back, shoulders, and triceps into the mat while lightly drawing the shoulder blades in [retraction] and down [depression]. This will create a lift in the chest and a slight back-bend in the thoracic spine [spinal extension]. Continue rooting through the upper body as you press from the hips into the feet to lift the hips up and away from the floor.

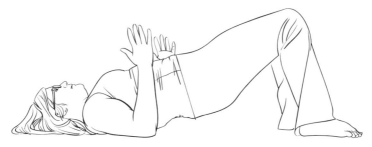

As the hips lift, you want to try and make sure that you don't feel as though you're pushing yourself backward on your mat. This usually happens when people try to lift too high and the fronts of the thighs [the quadriceps] get overly involved. You also want to be aware of any excess external rotation happening in the hips, which would present as the knees falling out to the sides and possibly the insteps of the feet lifting away from the floor. [Biomechanically, we would say that Bridge is a pose of extension: hip extension, which is the action of the glutes; spinal extension, which is the action of the spinal extensors; and shoulder extension, which is the action of the deltoid and triceps.]

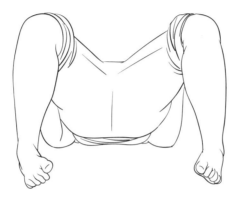

After three to ten breaths, soften through the glutes to lower the hips back down. Soften the upper body, straighten the arms, and maybe even straighten the legs on the floor, if that feels appropriate. Alternatively, you could slide blocks, a blanket, or a bolster under the knees. Notice the response from the body. What kinds of sensations are there? Are there any thoughts surrounding the sensations? Can you stay with the feeling of the sensations even while thinking is happening?

Legs Up the Wall

Start sitting next to the wall, with the feet flat on the floor and one hip against the wall. As you start to roll onto the back, swing the legs up and onto the wall, hence the name Legs Up the Wall, such that your body is perpendicular to the wall with your head farthest from it. Adjust the distance between your hips and the wall such that the spine can be in a neutral position, which ensures that the low spine is pressing into the floor and the pelvis is not rolling off the mat. The arms can rest beside the torso, or you can place the hands on the belly or ribs, whichever is most comfortable.

[We try to have participants in this posture for three to five minutes. That being said, not everyone's body is going to like it, so remind participants that they can come out of the pose at any time if it starts to feel uncomfortable or inappropriate.]

To make your way out of Legs Up the Wall, slide the feet down the wall, draw the knees in toward the chest, roll to one side, and then press yourself up to a seated position.

In yoga speak, we call Legs Up the Wall a restorative inversion. This posture has the strong potential to settle the body and calm the mind. That being said, there are a few things to keep in mind as far as modifications are concerned. If you notice someone's shoulders rolled away from the floor or neck craned, with the chin tilting toward the ceiling, try placing a folded blanket, approximately one to two inches thick, under their pelvis and slightly into the space of the low back. This will help the pelvis and low spine find a more neutral position and will potentially allow the shoulders and neck to also find a better position.

If the hips have to be away from the wall to find a neutral spine, the knees will likely hyperextend. This might cause discomfort in the backs of knees. There are two modifications for this. You can have participants place their feet flat on the wall with the knees bent, or tie a strap around the thighs just above the knee to help keep the knees from hyperextending. If the shoulders are still rounded and the neck craned even after adding a blanket or shifting the hips away from the wall so that the spine can find neutral, place a thinly folded blanket under the back of the head.

Group Dialogue: Debriefing Yoga Practice

Invite participants to sit at the front of their mats, and conduct a brief discussion about the practice. Encourage noticing by asking, "What showed up for you in that practice? Anyone notice striving or other impulses to push harder or to perform?" And finally, "Were you able to listen to what your body was telling you, or did your mind get hooked?"

Transition from the group dialogue to a brief perspective-taking meditation. It's helpful to set aside extra time for the home practice because the nutrition and eating discussion can take a lot of time. Furthermore, during this discussion, it's helpful to draw participants' attention to any escaping, avoiding, or controlling involved in their relationship with food, which can also take time. So, be mindful of how much time is spent in the debriefing and meditation.

Values and Vulnerabilities (Through the Eyes of a Loved One)

In this perspective-taking meditation, you'll encourage participants to slow down and see if they can picture the world from behind the eyes of someone close to them. While we encourage connecting with a personal value—someone who matters to each participant—we simultaneously encourage participants to make contact with a painful experience.

> I invite you to picture someone in your life with whom you've felt connected, perhaps someone who appreciated you, someone who saw some value in you. It could be a caregiver, such as a parent, or someone with a special interest in you, perhaps a friend, a partner, or a teacher. Picture someone who has really valued you.
>
> Take a moment to close your eyes and see if you can visualize this person. Picture them as vividly as possible. Take a moment to picture their face, noticing the details of their eyes and eyebrows. Let yourself see their hair, their lips, and their nose.
>
> What is the emotion on their face as they look at you?
>
> Try to really see them looking at you in this moment. And notice what that feels like for you as you look into their eyes and feel their connection.
>
> Now I invite you to slip your awareness out from behind your eyes and place it behind theirs, seeing yourself from behind their eyes. Seeing yourself

as someone whom they want to connect with, someone of value, someone who is appreciated.

What do you feel?

As you're feeling what they feel looking at you and seeing your eyes, take a breath and notice what that's like in your body.

Noticing the sensations of breath in your body. When you feel ready, bring some motion into your body, such as wiggling the fingers, rotating the wrists, rolling the shoulders up, back, and down, and moving the head from side to side.

End this exercise by instructing participants to break into groups of two and to share what they noticed. Give each participant two minutes to do this. Invite them to avoid sharing the content of what happened specifically in the meditation but instead to share about what it was like for them personally. Have them finish by sharing what they would have to get rid of or not care about anymore in order to no longer suffer.

Group Dialogue: Debriefing Values and Vulnerabilities

Invite participants to return to the larger group and share what they noticed. Some participants may choose to tell the story of what happened for them privately during the meditation, and how that manifested as something important. They may even explain how that important thing changed, perhaps becoming clearer as they discussed the content with their small-group partner. That's good, because the purpose of the debrief is to have them track specifically what they noticed and how that impacts them—a sort of second level of noticing.

Session Three Home Practice: Nutrition and Eating

For the session three home practice, we encourage participants to come into contact with thoughts, emotions, memories, and sensations that are linked with food in general and specific foods in particular. We provide participants a mindful eating script to practice at home, both as a way to transform their relationship with food and to provide another example of how mindful attention can increase our engagement with the world. If participants begin to discuss different types of diets or fads, or ask your opinions on what they should eat, redirect them. The goal of the at-home practice is not for them to get sucked into the content of specific food groups or diets, rather it's to pay more attention when consuming food or beverages. A common outcome of being more mindful of what we put in our bodies is a desire to change our dietary habits. If participants tell you they want to make significant changes to their eating habits following this week of mindful eating, encourage them to discuss any dietary changes with their doctor, particularly if they have medical conditions or are taking medications.

> In a moment, we're going to do a mindful eating exercise. I'm also going to give you a copy of the script so you can practice this exercise at home over the next week. The idea behind this practice is to slow down and connect to the process of eating while engaging all of your senses. What does the food look like? Does it have a smell? Can you hear it as you chew or swallow? Does it crackle or sizzle before you eat it? Is there a particular texture you associate with it? And finally, what does it taste like? We want you to approach food as if you're just now discovering it and want to pause and take a closer look.
>
> You don't have to eat like a slowly munching panda, or place your fork down between each bite, or be that person who moans when they eat. Though we may purposely exaggerate slowness in this exercise, the message we want to send is that even when you're pressed for time, you have an opportunity to notice what is happening as you consume food or beverage. Similar to yoga, this way of eating is simply another active form of paying attention. Because we eat and drink multiple times every day, we're often very distracted when we do so, so being mindful of these activities is a great way to practice noticing—and to actually enjoy and taste—the food we're eating, instead of simply scarfing it down.
>
> Read through the Mindful Eating Script and give it a go the next time you sit down, stand at the sink, or hunch over your desk to eat. You can do this practice with any food, snack, or meal.

Encourage participants to practice the script at home and to keep a Mindful Eating Log in which they track when they practice mindful eating and what their experience was like. We provided a sample log after the Mindful Eating Script, and you can download both these forms at http://www.newharbinger.com/42358.

Mindful Eating Script

1. Take the food and hold it (or the plate it is on) in your hand. Is it cool, neutral in temperature, or warm to the touch? Is it soft or firm?

2. Look at the food closely. Is it uniform in color? Uneven in shape or color? Flawed or unflawed? Is there a noticeable pattern or design on it?

3. Does the food make any sound as you hold it or move it between your fingers?

4. Examine the food as if you've never encountered it before. Wonder about it. What is it? Where did it come from? How was it made or grown?

5. Now smell the food. Does it have a scent, or is it odorless?

6. Notice any urges to eat it. Do you have any sense of impatience? What about thoughts, feelings, or desires?

7. Be aware of your conscious decision to eat this food. Note any thoughts or feelings. Do you feel any sense of excitement?

8. Now put the food in your mouth and let it rest on your tongue. What does it taste like before you bite down? What is the texture like? How does it feel on your tongue? Is it rough or smooth? Does it taste sweet or salty?

9. Now bite into the food. Chew it slowly. How does the flavor change? Does it make a sound as you bite into it? Is the texture the same?

10. Does this food evoke any feelings or memories? Practice being aware of the distinction between the sensations in the moment and all the thoughts and feelings evoked by the act of eating.

11. After swallowing, pause to notice any changes in the sensations of hunger or your appetite.

12. Once you've finished eating the food, pause and reflect on the experience. Notice any thoughts of wanting more or any feelings of having enough. What else can you be aware of before your transition to your next activity?

Mindful Eating Log

	Date	Time	Food	What did you notice?
Monday				
Tuesday				
Wednesday				
Thursday				
Friday				
Saturday				
Sunday				

Ending Savasana: Consciousness in Motion

This final relaxation pose winds down the third session of MYACT and offers one last meditation on perspective taking. Have participants find Savasana on their mats.

Let's take a breath on purpose, giving ourselves an extra deep inhale. On your exhale, breathe all the way out.

As you're here in this room surrounded by other people who have come to this space to take an active role in improving their life, just breathe in the fact that the people here have really showed up to being vulnerable, bringing their whole self to this room.

I invite you to picture yourself standing at the bank of a river. Pause to notice the sensory details—really be there behind your eyes. Notice the color of the water, and its shape as it pushes past you.

Long before you stood here at this bank, the river was here, carving its pathway through the land, finding its way to the ocean, digging lakes, eroding rock, and carrying sand. This water will continue to be here long after you and I have left this planet, continuing to rise from its source and make its way to the ocean.

Pause to reflect on the long history of suffering on this planet, the suffering that took place before you or any other person in this room was here. And notice what it's like to also recognize that this suffering will continue long after we've all left. Whatever shows up, just breathe it in.

And before we end our session and engage in our good-bye ritual, I'd like to invite you to find some stillness in this room, in this moment, as we lay in Savasana, breathing in our own histories, our own suffering, and the history of suffering that the peoples of this planet have endured. Breathing in the ongoing flow of history and suffering. Pause to witness it, and breathe.

Coming back to this room, feel the weight of your body on your mat, supported by the earth. Bring some motion into the body, such as a wiggle of the fingers or a rotation of the wrists. Bring some motion into the toes and the ankles. Move the head gently from side to side. And when you feel ready, rolling to your right, using the left arm to raise yourself up, come to be seated at the front of your mat to begin our good-bye ritual.

Once all participants are seated at the top of their mat, end this third session of MYACT as you ended session one, with chanting, sharing appreciations, and a closing posture.

Working with Individuals

- Rather than use the Escape, Avoidance, and Control Checklist, you may want to have a more fluid conversation with your client. If a client is struggling to identify avoidance strategies, the checklist may come in handy for providing suggestions.

- If a discussion on nutrition and dieting is not appropriate for your setting, you may choose to do a mindful eating exercise in session or have the client complete it as homework as another way to practice incorporating mindfulness into everyday life.

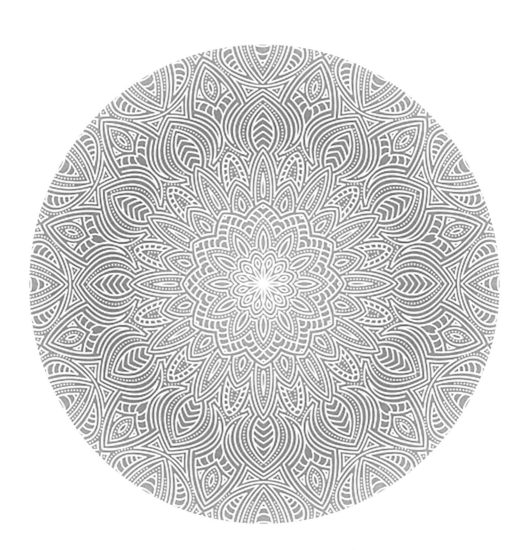

Karma

The fourth session of MYACT focuses on *karma*, the Sanskrit word for "action" that is interpreted in the Vedic traditions to mean "Through your actions you create your life." Practitioners of the Vedic perspective believe in free will, but the tradition implies that to claim free will, one must interrupt the patterned behaviors (samskāras) that are problematic—those that lead to attachment and more suffering. ACT adds a brand-new slant to this yogic practice by teaching practitioners to engage life guided by their unique values. ACT empowers practitioners to choose the qualities they wish to be guided by, and in yoga, they spontaneously take action. This action is not focused on the immediate outcome of what happens but rather on what keeps us connected with what matters most, so we can live life well in the long run.

Beginning Meditation: Allowing Your Pain In

We ended our last session by coming in contact with the ongoing flow of experience. In the same way that we can stand at the bank of a river, observing its ongoing flow and perceiving its history before us and its future after us, we can bring suffering into our awareness.

Today, in our fourth session, I invite you to let your pain in. When we get hooked by our pain, the mind makes fast work of attempts to escape, avoid, or control. This meditation is an invitation to breathe your pain in, letting it be in this room with us. Your challenge is to welcome your pain, to welcome the pain of others here in this room. Please find yourself in Savasana.

Settling into your body, take a breath on purpose.

Honor the stillness in your body. Seek it out and be with it. Notice cool air as you inhale, and slightly warmer air as you exhale. See if you can notice the specific details of cool air as you inhale and warm air as you exhale.

And shift your awareness away from the breath to your history. Acknowledging times in your life when you struggled, when your own thoughts and feelings about yourself were painful for you. Maybe these are situations when your mind told you that you're not good enough or that you're a failure, or maybe when your mind tried to problem solve how you could be better but only made you feel worse. And see yourself in one of those situations. And if your mind bounces around, that's okay. Allow yourself to hit that instant replay on a particularly painful moment and see your face there. What does the look on your face look like? How about the shape of your eyes? What is the look in your eyes like? However old this memory may be, as you breathe here, see if you can acknowledge the length of time this pain has followed you around in your life.

And wherever your mind takes you, breathe here and reach back even further in time, to earlier times when you struggled with this pain. Times when you knew what this pain cost you, the toll that you've paid in life, the loss, the impact…breathe that history in. And imagine that you can see an even younger version of yourself struggling with this pain. Perhaps in your early teenage years, or in your early adolescence. Picture yourself suffering with this in your early adolescence. Picture your face suffering with this. And really take in that image. See your face in that hardest moment for you. Know that the pain the adolescent you is experiencing is the same pain you know now; the struggles that this you is battling are the same struggles you know now.

And go back further still, to the youngest version of yourself that you can recall when this pain showed up in your life. Go back to the earliest memory you have of struggling with this pain, and see that younger version of you. Perhaps see a place where the younger you struggled with this. Whether it be at home, with family, in a classroom, or on a playground, really picture this younger you there. Who were you with? Who else could you see? Perhaps you were by yourself. Picture the clothing you were wearing. The color of your hair. The shape of your face. And how does this younger version of you who is suffering hold their body? What posture do they take?

And as you are here looking back into that history, look down into the face of the younger you, as if you could be present with them now. Look into their eyes. Take a breath. Perhaps you can see something in their eyes that other people can't see. Imagine that you could reach out, make a gesture toward this younger you, this child who suffers. Maybe reaching out, just adopting a gesture that feels right, maybe holding them, hugging them, touching their face, feeling their warmth. And as you reach for them, simply offering them some words of validation. Whether it's "I know" or "I'm here," let them know that they are not alone. Maybe you can just say, "I see your hurt." When they look up into your eyes, imagine that they can feel your connection and your warmth, that you understand their hurt, that your hurt is their hurt, and that you're not a stranger to their pain.

And breathe here. Notice what it's like to be in this moment. What it could mean to this child that you were willing to slow down into this moment to see their hurt and to acknowledge it. And if you were to offer some last parting words that could carry them forward, what might those parting words be? Just listen to your heart as it communicates this message to them. Speak softly, speak slowly.

Take a breath. And just gently draw back, allowing yourself to disconnect from them. Drawing your body back. Breathe here and allow the image to pass. Returning to the sensations of your breath, feel it in your body. Allowing all the images we've evoked in this exercise to just drift, like water running past you. Notice the sound of my voice, and bring some motion into your body. Wiggle the fingers. Rotate the wrists. And just allow yourself to come to some rest in this moment, totally present with what you feel. Feeling the emotional qualities that show up for you. Noticing the coolness of each inhalation, the warmth of each exhalation. Gently allow yourself to become aware of the room that you're in, the temperature of the air on your skin.

Group Dialogue: Debriefing Beginning Meditation

After ending Savasana, invite participants to return to the larger group. Ask each participant to share, in a word, their experience of the meditation. Participants often struggle to show themselves love, acceptance, and compassion but find it easy to share them with their younger self. The meditation may evoke emotions such as anger or deep sadness for the younger self. That's okay. Encourage participants to show up and notice whatever their experience is.

Group Dialogue: Debriefing Home Practice

Encourage each participant to reflect on their MYACT practice over the past week and share what they noticed. The debriefing of the home practice is an opportunity for participants to talk about how the home practice went, to reinforce their engagement in new behaviors, and to troubleshoot problems that may have arisen. Here are some prompts to help with this:

Before we move on, how did everyone feel after they went home last week?

Did you have any difficulty or success practicing mindful eating?

How was it to do this practice?

What did you notice while doing it?

Did you commit yourself to any values-based behaviors this week?

Values Authorship

In this exercise, you'll define four life domains (connect, accept, let go, grow) and ask participants to share an example for each one that that they can purposefully choose to make their life about. You'll then have participants transition into groups of two, in which they'll help each other author and record their values in each of the four domains. We recommend that you hand out a clipboard with a pen and one Connect, Accept, Let Go, Grow worksheet to each participant. You can download the worksheet, along with other accessories for this book, at http://www.newharbinger.com/42358. As we indicate in the following sections, these four life domains map onto the four quadrants of the life map.

Connect

Relationships are work, and rarely does society offer practical, real-world advice for what to do when relationships present challenges or people struggle to stay connected. The connect domain is what it sounds like: it's the life domain in which you consider who and what you wish to forge new or deeper connections with. These values are found in the bottom-right quadrant of the life map. Apart from insisting that each participant identify one example of who or what (a quality, or a noun such as "nature") they value, be sure to ask why what they value matters: "What would connection with this person or this quality mean to you?"

Accept

Participants often ask us what they can do about their painful private experiences, and we believe the domain of acceptance quickly cuts to the core of what they should do. Have them identify a painful private experience that they can't escape or permanently delete. This is what they will work to accept, or make peace with, in order to stop struggling and start living a better life. We like the "make peace with" language because the word "accept" can be difficult for some participants, especially those with a history of being told to "get over" their experiences. These painful private experiences are found in the bottom-left quadrant of the life map.

Let Go

Letting go is about identifying the problematic behaviors we tend to engage in to escape, avoid, or control painful private experiences and choosing to engage in these behaviors less often. These behaviors are found in the top-left quadrant of the life map.

Grow

Focusing on behaviors we want to grow in our lives is about improving or maintaining what matters most. We feel it important to include the word "maintain" because participants may already engage in valuable behaviors that they take for granted. The word drives this point home and hopefully ensures that the behaviors that are already working persist. Challenge participants by asking them, "In what ways do you want to grow in your life? What things are you already doing that you want to nurture in your life?" The behaviors, or committed actions, of this domain are found in the top-right quadrant of the life map.

Group Dialogue: Debriefing Values Authorship

Allow each participant at least five minutes in their groups of two before bringing the larger group back together and asking participants to share what they noticed in the exercise. We transition from this exercise into the session's yoga practice by encouraging participants to pay attention to their values to see how congruent their yoga practice is with these values.

Yoga Is Valuing

Take a few moments to translate for participants how the practice of yoga can be a way of exploring one's values. Consider exploring what their values are around the yoga practice itself. Common answers include health, exercise, and challenging oneself. From this perspective, showing up to a yoga practice with the aim of sweating, working hard, or simply getting a good workout might be in line with a person's values; however, there might also be times when pushing harder or staying in a pose longer can be about fusing with unhelpful, rigid rules. A participant may become stuck on thoughts such as *I have to stay in this pose as long as I did last time or as long as everyone else holds it!*

Talk to participants about focusing on the motivation behind their actions, not the actions themselves, because the same movement or yoga pose can be both about living one's values and control and avoidance. For one person, staying in a pose longer can be

Connect, Accept, Let Go, Grow

Answer the questions below, asking yourself if what you're writing is important in your life. Will moving toward these goals help you to be the person you want to be?

1. Connect

   - Who or what in my life do I choose to forge a new or deeper connection with?

   _____

   _____

2. Accept

   - What painful experiences in my life do I choose to accept or make peace with?

   _____

   _____

3. Let Go

   - What problematic behaviors do I want to engage in less often in my life?

   _____

   _____

4. Grow

   - What behaviors do I want to grow in my life to improve or maintain who and what are important to me?

   _____

   _____

Committing to Growth

Pick one response from each question to begin working toward. You will use the Daily Commitment Questions Recording Form to track your success in connecting with what matters to you, accepting painful experiences, letting go of problematic behaviors, and growing behaviors that move you toward the life you want to live.

I commit to begin working toward:

Connecting with _____

Accepting _____

Letting go of _____

Growing _____

about moving toward a value of self-improvement, whereas for another person, it may be a way to escape or avoid painful thoughts. Ask participants to check in with their values as they move and breathe. Remind them to align their physical practice with what they wish to be about in that moment.

Sometimes we frame this concept with the phrase "attention, intention, action." We've taught participants how to pay deeper attention to what's happening moment to moment (attention) and helped them connect with and even name who and what are important to them. Now we want to orient them in the direction of those values. "Intention is everything" is a colloquialism that applies here. Intention is really just the direction we're pointing ourselves in. Our goal in attending to our actions and identifying our values ourselves is to intentionally take steps toward our values. If we can notice, then we have a higher likelihood of choosing our values in that moment. Upon taking that first step, we come back to attention, and the cycle starts again: attention, intention, action. This question can be very valuable during this yoga practice: "Is how you're approaching this posture helping you move closer to who and what are important to you?"

As far as the movements in this session are concerned, try to reinforce the value of slow, intentional movement and smooth breathing. When we consciously practice good movement patterns (behaviors) and reinforce those patterns as often as we can, the body starts to execute the patterns without as much conscious effort. Over time, it becomes easier to check in with ourselves in each moment to see in which direction we're stepping and to adjust accordingly.

You'll now conduct the fourth yoga sequence, comprising the following practices:

- Cat and Cow and Child's Pose Flow

- Standing Half-Sun Salutation

- Tree

- Warrior 3

- Group Tree

Cat and Cow and Child's Pose Flow

Start in Table. As you connect to the feel—pace, depth, length, fluidity—of your breath, begin to move through four rounds of Cat and Cow tilts. [Refer to session two.]

After rounding the spine and dropping the head into Cat, briefly shift the hips back toward the heels, coming into Child's Pose. The following inhale brings you back up through Table and into Cow. The exhale moves you through Cat and back to Child's Pose.

It's okay if the hips and heels don't touch during Child's Pose, especially if doing so creates any stress in the knees, low back, or shoulders. Also, as you shift back, gently press from the shoulders and armpits down into the hands, not as though you're using the arms to push the hips back, but just to maintain some integrity in the shoulders and to encourage upward rotation, a necessary shoulder blade movement when the arms move into flexion.

Move through five to ten rounds at your own pace with smooth, easy breathing.

Standing Half-Sun Salutation

Begin standing at the front of your mat with your feet hip-width apart.

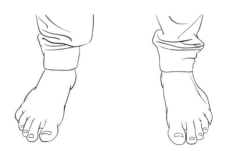

Bring the hands to heart center, deepening and lengthening the breath. In this pose, we use the breath to keep our pace as we move. The breath becomes like a metronome for our movements. On an exhale, lower your arms to your sides. With a slow inhale, sweep the arms forward and up toward the ceiling.

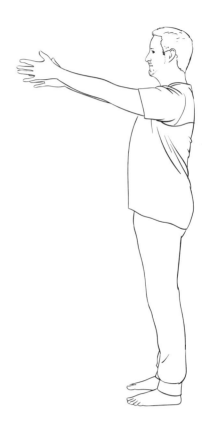

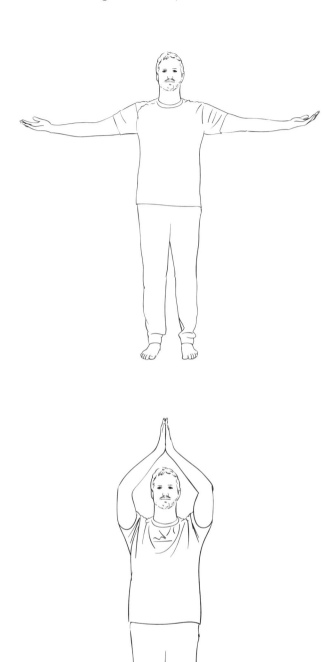

As the arms come overhead, bring the palms together. As you exhale, slide your hands down to heart center. Again, with a slow inhale, sweep the arms forward and up, noticing how that feels in your body. Again, the palms of the hands come together overhead, and with an exhale, slide the hands back to heart center. One more time, as you inhale deeply, the arms sweep forward and up. Really notice how that feels in your body. And as you exhale, bring the hands back to heart center. This time, as you inhale, sweep the arms sideways and up toward the ceiling, again noticing how this movement feels in your body.

As the palms of the hands come together overhead, exhale to slide the hands down to heart center. Do this movement two more times with your breath. Next, from the hands at heart center, and keeping the palms together, inhale to move the arms straight up toward the ceiling.

Keeping the palms together, exhale and slide the hands down to heart center, noticing how this particular movement feels in your body. Try this movement two more times. At the end of the final round, as the hands come to rest at heart center, take a moment to notice which movement felt best for you, whether it was the arms sweeping forward and up, sideways and up, or straight up. I recommend that you use whichever one felt best for the rest of your Standing Half-Sun Salutations.

Still standing at the front of your mat, connecting to the feeling of your breath moving in and moving out, inhale to reach the arms up toward the ceiling.

As you reach up, there is the option to take your gaze toward the hands, but if this irritates the neck, feel free to keep your gaze forward, allowing the neck to remain neutral and relaxed. As you exhale, begin to tilt the pelvis forward as you start to move into Standing Forward Fold.

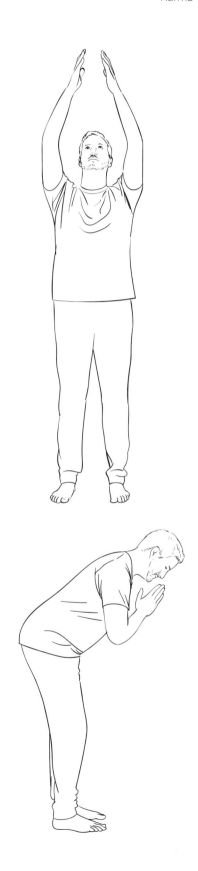

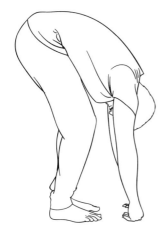

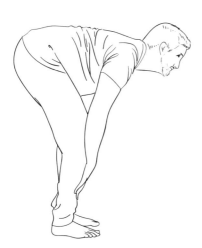

As the body folds forward, try to feel that the movement starts at the pelvis so that you aren't just rounding your spine as you fold forward. Ideally, the spine stays long until the pelvis can't tilt forward anymore, and then the spine begins to round. As you're coming into your Standing Forward Fold, it's also important to not lock your knees. They should remain bent slightly. When you find your Standing Forward Fold, have enough bend in the knees so that the low belly can rest on the upper thighs.

From there, keeping the knees bent, place your hands on your shins. As you inhale, contract the muscles in the back to lift and lengthen your spine.

As you lengthen the spine, draw the shoulder blades together toward the midline. On a slow exhale, allow the spine to round toward the legs. As you inhale, return back to a standing position as you lift the arms up.

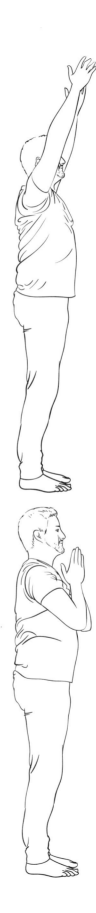

Exhale to bring the hands to heart center.

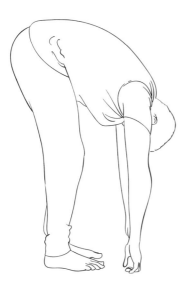

Just note that there is more than one way to come back to standing as far as your pelvis and spine are concerned. We're not trying to "rag doll" the spine up to standing, which has the potential to overstress the spine and the discs that sit between each vertebra.

Instead, our approach utilizes more of the hip strength, along with spinal strength, to bring you back up to standing while decreasing the stress on the spine. Here's a practice exercise to explore how to feel this difference in your body. Come into your Standing Forward Fold, with enough bend in the knees so the belly can rest on the upper thighs. Take the hands to the shins and inhale to lengthen the spine and open the chest by drawing the shoulder blades together. Pause here in this flat-back position for an exhale. On your next inhale, maintain this long spine as you use the hips to bring yourself up to vertical. Try this a few more times to familiarize yourself with the movement.

When you're first learning Standing Half-Sun Salutation, it's okay if you add this little exercise to the middle of the sequence to help yourself learn the movement. Once you've mastered the movement of how to come back up properly, when you inhale to come back up to standing, the first half of the inhale is used to lift and lengthen the spine, and the second half of the inhale is for utilizing the hips to bring you back up to vertical as you lift the arms overhead.

After finishing with Standing Half-Sun Salutation, we focus on balancing postures. These postures require participants to attend to small movements in their body and to where their body is in relation to the room and others. Encourage them to have patience and flexibility around what they're asking their body to do. There will be many modifications throughout this practice, and many people falling out of balance. Acknowledge this and encourage participants to focus on the process of finding balance rather than landing a certain posture.

Tree

Start standing with your feet together. It's better to start Tree with the feet together so that you can more easily transfer the load onto one foot without falling over.

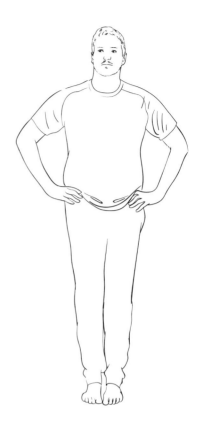

For the first, and easiest, variation, keep the left foot flat on the floor and the hips square. Externally rotate the right leg out and bend that knee slightly to bring the toes to the floor.

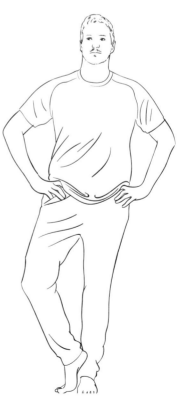

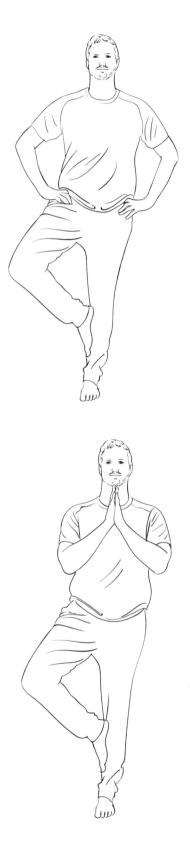

In this variation, you can use the right toes on the floor to assist with balance. [We always say, "It's better to practice balancing than to practice falling over."] If you feel that you don't need the toes on the floor to maintain balance, the next option is to slide the foot up onto the calf.

You can keep the hands on the hips or bring them to heart center.

As you're balancing, really do your best to stay relaxed in your breathing. When we feel unsteady or off-balance, we have a natural tendency to get rigid and hold our breath. Can you soften into the imbalance, accept the inherent wobbliness of the posture, and learn to work with the wobbling instead of trying to control it? [The imagery we like to use in any standing balance posture is that of a tightrope walker. The tightrope walker is constantly settling into their breathing and taking in information from the environment—the rope under their feet, any mild or strong breeze that might arise, and so on. They're working "with" what is arising instead of trying to deny or control it. They practice meeting the moment as it arises.]

Stay here balancing for as long as the breath can stay smooth. When you can no longer support the posture with good breathing, switch to the other side. When you shift to the opposite leg, remember that your body and balance will be different. It's important to recognize that you do not have a good leg or a bad leg. The reality is that you have a leg with more stability and a leg with less stability. If it seems as though even standing on one foot with the opposite toes on the floor for help is too difficult, you always have the option to use a wall or a chair for help, using either as much as it's needed to maintain the stance.

Warrior 3

Start standing with the feet together. Having the feet together allows for a slightly easier transition of weight when moving into balancing postures. Have the arms down at your sides. Shift your weight onto the right foot, lifting the left foot slightly away from the floor while keeping that leg straight. Begin to hinge at the right hip, tilting the pelvis forward over the right thigh bone [femur]. As the pelvis tilts forward, the spine stays neutral and also begins to move forward. At the same time, the left leg begins to travel back in space. The spine and the left leg should stay in one long line, so hinge only as far as that remains possible. You want to think of Warrior 3 as a seesaw or a teeter-totter; the right hip is the fulcrum and everything else moves around that particular axis.

When it's time to come out of the position, just as the pelvis moved us into it, the pelvis should bring us out. Everything from the left foot to the crown of the head stays in one long line.

Very common misalignments can arise as people get into this pose. Some people will naturally lead the movement with their spine instead of the pelvis, which ends with a pose that looks like an abdominal crunch, with a rounded upper spine. As the body is moving into position, others will stop the pelvis from moving relative to the femur, and the spine will keep going, which also presents as a shortening on the front side of the torso. This pose will end up looking like a sloppy capital *T*. Another common misalignment is when the pelvis can't tilt forward anymore, and the unsupported hip will begin to roll open to an unsquare position; for example, the left-hand side will get further away from the floor than the right-hand side. Yoga instructors commonly tell participants to just resquare the pelvis; however, we tend to back people up and get them to only move into the posture to the point that the hips can remain square. Remember, the goal is functional movement, not forcing the body into a position it can't handle without compensation or injury. It's also very important to watch out for participants who tend to lock the knees or hyperextend them. Guide them to bend the knees slightly.

Some variations of this posture include having the arms more out to the sides or toward the front of the mat. These both require more strength in the hips, core, low back, and shoulders. Other options include placing the hands on blocks or a wall for balance.

Group Tree

For Group Tree, participants will move into a circular formation, all facing in toward the center of the circle. Everyone will stand with their elbows close to their sides and bent so the lower portion of their arm is pointed up, left palm facing up and right palm facing down. Everyone in the group will then place their right palm down on the left palm of the person beside them.

> In this Group Tree, you'll choose whether to keep your toes on the floor or to place your foot on your calf. The point of this variation is balancing as a group, not challenging your own balance. It's about balancing your relationship with the people around you. As each of you finds your own variation of Tree, it's okay to communicate with the people beside you about how much pressure to place in their hands. It's also important to keep in mind that falling over is part of the process. One of the ways we get to know each other better is to communicate and to stumble and to communicate about how we stumble and then to work as a group to reestablish balance. Soften into your breathing, relax your shoulders, tell your partners what you need, and do your best to be open and receptive to what they need.

Group Dialogue: Debriefing Yoga Practice

Encourage each participant to sit at the front of their yoga mat in a comfortable seated posture: "Moving in your own time, find yourself seated at the front of your mat." Then debrief the practice with questions like these:

> What did you notice in that practice?

> What was important to you about the time you spent on the mat today?

> Did that or anything else surprise you?

> Noticing what was important, how did that impact your practice?

> How does it impact your perception of practicing?

> If the group is sheepish about answering the last question, sometimes we'll offer our own interpretation, saying, "I notice that what was important strengthens my resolve to be here, to do this work for myself, with you."

Commitment Questions

Building upon the values authorship exercise from earlier in the session, have participants return to their Connect, Accept, Let Go, Grow worksheets. Share an example of a commitment question and then transition the group to their groups of two and have them help each other write commitment questions for themselves on the worksheet.

Explain that each participant should have one commitment question for each of the four life domains (connect, accept, let go, grow). They should write their questions in the active voice, such as "Today did I do my best to…?" in order to place themselves at the center of the chain of action. They are, after all, the ones who either do or don't do the behaviors. These active questions discourage participants from blaming or excusing environmental cues, which are out of their control, for blocking or stopping a committed action. Here's an example of a commitment question for each domain:

Connect: Today, did I do my best to connect with my partner?

Accept: Today, did I do my best to make peace with the thought *I'm unlovable*?

Let go: Today, did I do my best to let go of always trying to appear like I'm okay—that is, not sharing vulnerability—when talking to my partner?

Grow: Today, did I do my best to improve my communication with my partner, such as by sending text messages throughout the day?

Session Four Home Practice: Daily Commitment Questions in Pairs

Pass out the Daily Commitment Questions Recording Forms, which are available for download at this book's website, http://www.newharbinger.com/42358. Instruct participants to reconvene their groups of two, in which they'll exchange phone numbers. Instruct them to agree to a time when they can talk by phone each evening between now and the next session, reading aloud their own commitment questions, one at a time, and scoring their own performance, from 0 (no effort at all) to 10 (maximum effort), related to the questions. Explain that they need not give feedback or ask exploratory questions of one another. This home practice is simply about keeping each other accountable to reflecting on the day's behavior and scoring one's performance.

Daily Commitment Questions Recording Form

Each day, score (from 0, no effort at all, to 10, maximum effort) your performance regarding the commitments you made for each domain on the Connect, Accept, Let Go, Grow worksheet. Ask yourself each of these questions before scoring yourself:

- *Did I do my best today to reduce a problematic behavior I want to **let go** of?*
- *Did I do my best today to **grow** my life toward improving or maintaining who and what are important to me?*
- *Did I do my best today to choose to **accept** or make peace with my painful experiences?*
- *Did I do my best today to **connect** to who and what are important to me?*

GROW

Sun	Mon	Tues	Wed	Thurs	Fri	Sat

CONNECT

Sun	Mon	Tues	Wed	Thurs	Fri	Sat

Paying attention

LET GO

Sun	Mon	Tues	Wed	Thurs	Fri	Sat

ACCEPT

Sun	Mon	Tues	Wed	Thurs	Fri	Sat

Ending Savasana or Seated Meditation: Loving-Kindness Meditation

Have participants find Savasana, or a seated position that is comfortable for them.

Take a breath on purpose. Feel the belly expand as you inhale and collapse as you exhale. Really feel that movement in your body.

Notice how the chest lifts as you breathe in and drops as you breathe out. See if you can focus your attention to stay with the movement of your breath in your body.

Inevitably, distractions will arise, whether it's a sound, a sensation like your nose itching, or tension in your body. Whenever distractions arise, notice them. They're inevitable. Come back to your breathing. Really pay attention to the sensations of your breath.

Take a moment to picture someone who is important to you, someone who depends on you or on whom you depend. Really picture them and say privately in your mind, or aloud, softly and slowly:

May you be happy.

May you be well.

May you have health.

May you know love.

May you find peace.

And breathe. Just notice anything that shows up for you. Allow their image to pass, come back to your breath, and now bring to mind someone whom you feel neutral toward, perhaps the clerk at a grocery store or coffee shop you see regularly, a coworker, or someone you see on your commute. Picture their face and say privately in your mind, or aloud, softly and slowly:

May you be happy.

May you be well.

May you have health.

May you know love.

May you find peace.

Now picture someone you have conflict with. Allow yourself to notice whatever shows up, even as I give you this instruction. Take a breath and see their face. Now in your mind, or aloud, say softly and slowly:

May you be happy.

May you be well.

May you have health.

May you know love.

May you find peace.

Regardless of what feelings, thoughts, or sensations arise for you, allow any of your reactions to be present as your awareness comes to include everything that you notice.

Finally, picture yourself. Really see yourself sitting here in this room. Picture your face. Share these words to yourself, or aloud, softly and slowly:

May I be happy.

May I be well.

May I have health.

May I know love.

May I find peace.

One last time, pause. Breathe in whatever shows up for you.

After making a visual check-in with each participant, end this fourth session of MYACT as you ended sessions one through three, with chanting, sharing appreciations, and a closing posture.

Working with Individuals

- Rather than using the Connect, Accept, Let Go, Grow worksheet, have a discussion with your client about these domains. You can even share your own examples, if doing so is functionally appropriate—that is, if it helps the client identify personal examples or models of being open and flexible.

- If you do decide to shorten the yoga practice, consider practicing Tree because it offers great opportunities for clients to pay attention to their motivations behind certain decisions (keeping their foot on the ground versus lifting it higher) and to be with feelings of discomfort and frustration as they struggle to maintain balance. It also highlights how efforts to control (maintain balance) are often unsuccessful and lead to the thing they were trying to avoid (falling over).

- To maintain the accountability for scoring the four commitment questions, ask your client to email you with their scores every day. Explain that they don't need to explain their scores, rather they simply need to report them.

SESSION FIVE

Svarūpa

In this fifth session of MYACT, we demonstrate how we can be freed from the tyranny of the mind, unhelpful rules, and attachment in order to live our essential nature as our true self. Connecting with the true self, realizing one's essential nature, is a Vedic concept called *svarūpa*, which Patañjali sought to expose through yoga. We encourage participants to play-fully engage their most difficult experiences rather than try to escape them or treat them with stoicism. This session is all about freedom, as loosening the hold pain has over us, reducing the strict governance of rules that painful feelings can embody, is the act of living free.

Importantly, we're not suggesting that participants live without pain. "Freedom" in our definition is living *with* pain, noticing how it impacts us, and choosing where we want to go in our lives. We carefully weave the word "relaxation" into these conversations about being free: "Could you lean into your pain and find relaxation there?" or "Feel whatever shows up and relax or soften into it." We're careful with our language to reduce the likelihood of pro-moting the idea that participants should have a dualistic relationship with pain. Pain and freedom are not mutually exclusive. Instead, we want participants to focus on being with their pain and finding some freedom from its control.

> **Pro Tip:** You can refer back to the discussion on hooks to make the point that pain and freedom are not mutually exclusive:
>
> When we bite a hook, we no longer have a choice over what happens next. It's as if that hook leads to an immediate, automatic avoidance reaction. Through opening up to our pain and noticing our hooks we can learn to create space between that hook and our automatic response. In that space lies freedom—the freedom to choose what to do next while in the presence of that pain, that hook.

Beginning Meditation: Go with It

This meditation shifts participants' attention in multiple ways. Incorporate into it sounds, sensations, and scents that you notice in the environment.

Take a breath on purpose, and as you exhale, gently close your eyes, if you are comfortable doing so, or look at a neutral place on the floor or in your lap. As you do this practice, if distractions arise or your mind tries to take you elsewhere, that's okay. That's what minds do. Simply notice that and turn your attention back to what I'm directing your attention to. This practice is all about noticing whatever shows up, going with it, and then directing our attention to where we want it.

Pause and listen to the sounds around you. What do you hear? Do you hear one sound or many sounds together? See if you can describe the sounds. Are they hard or soft, high or low, continuous or intermittent? Notice that you hear the sound. Are you the sound? Can you pinpoint where each sound is in relation to you? Notice that there is a difference between you and the sound. There is the sound and there is you to notice the sound.

[Invite people to listen to the sound of a noise you make.] Notice that you hear this sound. Notice that you are the one who hears this sound.

[Invite people to listen to the sound of another noise you make.] Notice that you hear this sound. Notice that you are the one who hears this sound.

Expand your attention out to the other people in the room with you. If you were hearing these sounds through their ears, would they sound the same? In what ways would the sounds be different?

Turning your attention back to your experience, shift your attention to your body. Feel where your body touches the chair. Imagine drawing an outline of where your body makes contact with the surfaces supporting it: the floor beneath you, or the back of a chair.

And as you're focusing on your body, slowly scan your body from the top of your head to the tips of your toes, bringing your attention to any emotions you experience. Maybe you feel quiet, restless, confused, irritated, or concerned. Feel where in your body you can experience emotions. Investigate the experience of the emotions. Are they strong or weak? Do they take up much space in your body, or little space? Are they in the forefront or in the background of your mind? Notice that you experience the emotions, that there is a you who is noticing emotions you experience. Notice that there is a difference between you and the emotions. There are the emotions, and there is you noticing them.

Shifting from your body to your mind, bring your attention to thoughts going through your mind. Notice your thoughts. How do you experience your thoughts? In images? As words? Loose strings of words or full sentences?

Are your thoughts moving slowly or racing? Notice that you notice your thoughts. Are you your thoughts? Notice the difference between you and your thoughts.

Now, allow your mind to drift to the background of your focus, and bring your attention to the tactile sensations underneath your fingers. Rub your hands along your pants or the mat beneath you, whatever is available to you. Notice what each sensation feels like. Is it rough or smooth, thick or thin, mixed textures or all one sensation? Are others experiencing the same sensations as you?

Notice that you are the one hearing sounds, noticing bodily sensations, experiencing emotions, and having thoughts. Whatever the form of your experience, you are there to notice it. You encompass your experiences. You are bigger than any of them.

Bring your attention to yourself in this room. Picture yourself in this room. Are you the image you make of yourself? Bring to mind the image of the person next to you, on your right. Is this person the image you make of him or her? Notice that someone in this room is making an image of you. Bring to mind an image of the person to your left. Be aware that someone in this room is making an image of you. Are you the image you made of the person on your left? Are you the image someone else made of you? Notice that you are here making an image. There is a difference between you and the image you make.

Pause and take a breath on purpose here, sink into this moment, and, when you're ready, in your own time, gently open your eyes and come back to the room.

Group Dialogue: Debriefing Home Practice

Ask each participant to reflect on their MYACT practice over the past week. Here's a list of questions that we've found useful to get the conversation going:

Before we move on, how did everyone feel after they went home last week?

Did you have any difficulty or success with the at-home practice?

What did you choose to connect with, accept, let go of, and grow?

How was it to do this practice?

What did you notice while doing it?

What was it like to share your rating with your partner every day?

Did you commit yourself to any values-based action this week?

Transition directly from the debrief into the three-part breath technique, which serves as a warm-up to the session's yoga practice. The technique encourages new ways of being with different experiences: "Our journey has revealed that escape from pain is not a workable agenda. Our logical conclusion is that if we're stuck with this yucky stuff, let's be playful with it and take it less seriously so we are free to choose where we want to go in our life."

Three-Part Breath Technique

Three-part breathing is a yogic breath that encourages participants to be present with their experience (or mindful).

Tune in to the natural movement of the breath, feeling where it goes without guidance. The beauty of the breath is that it was designed to move. Our job in prāṇāyāma, the practice of breathing, is simply to enhance what's already happening. Begin to add depth to your inhales and length to your exhales. At first, as you feel that deeper and longer breath moving through the body, just feel where the breath wants to move as you add some effort. Remember that we're not forcing the breath, we're simply guiding it. After a few deep breaths, noticing its movements, start to aim your inhales down into your belly. If it's helpful, place a hand or a block on the belly so that the breath is easier to feel. As you inhale into the belly, breathe in so that the belly rises naturally on the inhale.

This belly breath is the first of three parts. Stay with it for at least five more breaths. As you maintain an awareness of the belly rising and falling, start to expand your attention to include the back of your rib cage, the area just below your shoulder blades.

With your next inhale, breathe down into the belly and then guide that breath into the back of the ribs, followed by a slow, smooth breath out. Breathing into the back of the ribs is the second of three parts. Stay with this two-part breath for at least five more rounds. As you practice these first two parts, expand your attention to include the area just below your collarbones.

With your next inhale, breathe down into the belly, then move that breath into the back of the ribs, and finally breathe up into the chest, toward the collarbones. This is the full three-part breath. If it's difficult to feel the breath in the chest, you might place a hand near the collarbones. As you explore breathing up toward the collarbones, try to notice if the throat, the muscles around the neck, and the muscles around the shoulders are getting involved or activating. You want the neck and shoulders to remain soft, so do your best to direct your breath only as much as allows this. Trying to breathe with the muscles around the neck is what we call stress breath.

As you're practicing this three-part breath, one option is to pause briefly between each phase of the breath. Start breathing into the belly and add a brief pause, just a second. Breathe into the back ribs and pause. Breathe up to the collarbones and pause. Breathe out slowly and smoothly. Inhale into the belly and pause, into the ribs and pause, and into the chest and pause. Exhale slow and easy.

If you find that adding the pauses creates too much confusion or even symptoms of anxiety, just let go of the pauses and return to the basic three-part breath. The pauses are something that you might have to work up to. After a few more rounds of three-part breathing, continue to maintain the depth and the length of each breath, but start to release the directing. Once you let go of this aiming, notice how the deep breath feels. Is it moving differently than when you first started? Is the breath moving in areas that you didn't notice before? Do you notice anything different in regard to the mind or thinking?

Pause and debrief with participants, asking them to share what thoughts came up for them. Ask them if the difficult thoughts that they often struggle with outside of session came up during the exercise.

Self-Disclosure Card Shuffle

For this group exercise, give each participant a blank note card and a pen. Instruct them to take a moment to write something painful that they've struggled with, either currently or historically. Tell them to write a few sentences about how they've suffered, and what this struggle has cost them in life emotionally and interpersonally. What have they done as a result of this struggle? Be sure to instruct them to keep the cards anonymous; they shouldn't include names or any identifying details. You, too, will participate in this activity, disclosing something painful you have struggled with and describing what it has cost you. Here's an example:

I'm worried that I won't be loved by important people in my life. When I was a baby, my parents were young and gave me up for adoption because they couldn't take care of me properly. I spent a while in an orphanage and was later adopted. When I was older, I tried to have a relationship with my biological family, but after meeting me, they didn't want to talk to me anymore. Today, I struggle with this because I believe people who are supposed to love me don't. This has a cost in my interpersonal relationships. I try hard to make people happy, and if something doesn't go well, I blame myself. It's exhausting to try and make everyone else happy while simultaneously fearing that they will ultimately leave me.

Allot five minutes or so for participants to write on their cards. Upon completion, have them turn their cards in, adding your own to the pile, and then shuffle and redistribute them. You should get a card as well. Tell them that it's okay if they receive their own card. Have each participant, one by one, read the card aloud.

Group Dialogue: Debriefing Self-Disclosure Card Shuffle

After all cards have been read, go around the group and ask each participant to describe, in a word or two, what they are feeling. You should also share what you feel in the moment. Then collect the cards and prompt the group to share what they noticed: "Thank you for participating. What did you notice?"

You can use additional prompts, such as "What was it like to hear someone else read your card?" and "How did hearing these cards read aloud impact the way you think or feel about the things you struggle with?" Often they'll share how they don't feel as alone now because they realize that everyone is struggling with something, or they report feeling more connected to the group members.

Yoga Is Freedom

Being flexible in the presence of painful experiences sounds like a great concept, and it largely remains just that, a concept—an idea that is forgotten when the proverbial shit hits the fan. Flexibility stays a concept until you work at the edges of your comfort zone in the presence of pain, learning to find your true nature and shaping and reinforcing that repertoire rather than reverting to old hooked behaviors. In the following yoga practice, participants will come into contact with the felt experience of flexibly approaching discomfort with an aim to be free, so they can choose how they handle the discomfort.

Of course, encourage participants not to try and just push through physical pain, but rather encourage presence in the face of whatever arises. If participants begin to feel physical discomfort or even pain, we often tell them that it's not a serious problem. It's just the body telling them that something is up. It's the body's way of trying to get your attention, especially if you've overlooked subtle signs of pain. When we turn toward our pain and suffering, more options become available. This is not true of attempts to avoid, escape, or control our pain. This idea is described well in Yoga Sūtra 2.16: "*Heyam dukkam anagatam*," or "Through practice, future suffering can be alleviated." Our ability to stay present even in the face of discomfort is how we step toward freedom.

You'll now conduct the fifth yoga sequence, comprising the following practices:

- Standing Half-Sun Salutation (continuous)

- Linking Warrior 1, Warrior 2, Triangle, and Side Angle

- Supported Fish

- Supported Forward Fold

Standing Half-Sun Salutation (Continuous)

Have the group do Standing Half-Sun Salutations, as described in session four, one right after the other to create continuous movement. We recommend three to ten rounds for this warm-up, depending on the ability of the group and how long the practice period will be.

Linking Warrior 1, Warrior 2, Triangle, and Side Angle

In a style of yoga known as ashtanga-vinyasa, usually described as a practice of linking breath and movement, it is common to have one posture flow into another, with the breath serving as a kind of metronome to maintain pace and smoothness of movement. This is what we'll do in this flow with Warrior 1, Warrior 2, Triangle, and Side Angle. It's important to mention that the flow is not about keeping up with the people around you. We often say, "Your breath is your pace. You don't need to breathe or move like the people around you." When participants are first learning a flow like this, you might keep them in each pose for a breath or two before transitioning to the next one. But we encourage you to move yourself and participants in the direction of syncing every movement within the flow with the pattern of the breath, which happens fairly effortlessly with poses like Sun Salutation.

Stand at the top of your mat in Mountain. On an exhale, step the right leg back, finding your Warrior 1 stance, with the arms down at your sides or hands on the hips. On an inhale, sweep the arms up toward the ceiling.

On an exhale, transition into Warrior 2. Keeping the front leg fixed, turn the pelvis to face more toward the right side of your mat, with the back foot roughly parallel to the back of your mat. Bring the arms parallel to the floor with the palms face down, and rotate the head to look toward the left hand, if that feels appropriate.

Moving into Triangle, on an inhale, straighten the left knee without locking the joint, and on an exhale, begin to tilt the pelvis laterally toward the left heel, bringing the left hand onto whatever feels comfortable—the thigh, the shin, a block, or maybe even a chair—while the right arm gently reaches up to the ceiling. If the neck allows it, take the gaze to the right hand. On an inhale, staying grounded through the feet, bring the pelvis and spine back up to vertical. Just as we moved the pelvis to come into Triangle, we want to lead with the pelvis to come out of the pose.

On an exhale, rebend the left knee, coming back to Warrior 2. Inhale here, and on the exhale, begin to tilt the pelvis laterally to move into Side Angle, bringing the left arm to wherever is comfortable, such as the forearm or hand on the thigh. The right arm might either move straight out from the right shoulder or come up more beside the right ear. On an inhale, come back to Warrior 2. Exhale to bring the hands to heart center.

On an inhale, step the right foot forward to the front of the mat. Take a moment to pause. Feel how the body and breath are responding. Notice any thoughts or feelings that might be arising.

Do the same flow on the other side. You might also move participants through this sequence two to five times per side. The option to stay in each movement for a breath or two is always available. It's crucial for participants to know that as they're doing this flow, their legs might start to fatigue. If that's the case, they can always shorten the distance between the feet, a stance that requires less strength and stamina. As with any form of movement or exercise, the more people do it (without overdoing it), the stronger, more stable, and coordinated they'll become, which will then allow them to maintain a longer stance for longer durations.

Earlier, we stated that we'd encourage you to move yourself and participants in the direction of syncing every movement within the flow with the pattern of breath. Verbally, this syncing would sound like this:

From standing at the front of your mat, take a few moments to connect to the length, depth, and pace of your breath. This breath will act as a sort of metronome for movement. On an exhale, step the right leg back, finding Warrior 1. As you inhale, reach the arms up. As you exhale, slowly transition to Warrior 2, pelvis more open and arms parallel to the floor. Inhale to straighten the left leg without locking the knee. Exhale and tilt the pelvis toward the front heel, coming into Triangle. While keeping the legs straight, inhale to bring the spine and pelvis back up to neutral. Exhale and bend the left knee into Warrior 2. Pause in Warrior 2 for an inhale. Exhale and tilt the pelvis toward the front heel, coming into Side Angle. Inhale to come back up to Warrior 2. Exhale and bring the hands to heart center. Inhale to step back to the front of your mat.

The ability to do the above vinyasa sequence takes time and practice, not only to get to know the forms and movements of each posture and how they flow together but also to learn how to move with the breath. Start slow and take your time. It's within the slowness that our attention is more efficient. We pay more attention to the pace of breath, to the accuracy of our movements, to what thoughts and feelings might arise about the movements, to our ability to do them, and to our breathing.

When we teach this sequence to beginners, we often do visualization work. For example, when participants are in Warrior 1, we'll invite them to close their eyes and visualize what the transition from Warrior 1 to Warrior 2 would look like. What changes about the legs? What changes happen around the pelvis? Where do the arms go? What does the neck do? After a moment of visualization, they practice making that transition happen in the body. Having them imagine themselves practicing these transitions in their minds before connecting with them in their body is a great way to bring perspective taking into asana practice.

After you've completed the flow portion of this yoga practice, you're going to lead participants through a couple of poses of restorative yoga, an asana practice that relies on props to help create, align, and support the positions. (Legs up the Wall, which we described in session three, usually sits under this umbrella.) A focus of restorative practice is to have each posture feel comfortable and supported. We want to be able to relax into each pose, which helps calm the nervous system and, from a yogic perspective, restores, renews, and brings clarity to the body and mind.

Supported Fish

For Supported Fish, you'll need either two blocks or a blanket. If using yoga blocks, place one at its lowest height, horizontally across the mat, and the second block slightly behind that on its second-highest height toward the top of the mat. When you lay down on top of the blocks, the first block should sit beneath the shoulder blades to help lift the chest, broaden the collarbones, and open the front of the shoulders. The second block is to support the back of the head, inviting the back of the neck to lengthen.

If you're using a blanket, roll it into a relatively tight cylinder and place it parallel to the long edge of the mat. Lie down on the blanket in such a way that its lower end sits beneath the mid-upper back [thoracic vertebrae eight through ten], and the rest of it runs up the length of the spine and supports the head.

Whether using blocks or a blanket, the legs can be in any comfortable position: straight and relaxed, feet flat on the floor, or cross-legged.

You can have participants stay here for one to four minutes, depending on time and how their body is responding to the position. In restorative postures, we don't want participants hanging in there and trying to convince themselves that they can put up with or manage pain or discomfort. Comfort is key.

Supported Forward Fold

For Supported Forward Fold, you'll need three to four blocks, a blanket, a stack of pillows, or a folding chair. Start in a seated position with the legs straight. You might prefer to have your hips elevated on a block with a rolled-up blanket under the knees for support and comfort. With the blocks, pillows, or folding chair in front of you, fold forward primarily from the hips, but allow the spine to round slightly if it feels appropriate and doesn't place too much pressure on the lower spine. One variation is simply to place the hands out on the floor in front to support the upper body. Another variation is to rest the head on blocks or stacked pillows. This creates what is known as a closed-chain position, which allows the neck and spinal muscle to soften more easily. The last variation is to rest the forehead on the seat of a chair, perhaps with the arms up.

As with Supported Fish, keep participants in this pose for one to four minutes. However, the same guidelines apply. Participants shouldn't move into a painful position. If, after reducing the depth of the fold, pain or discomfort persist, have them try adjusting their props. Adjusting a prop an inch can be the difference between discomfort and absolutely blissful relaxation.

Group Dialogue: Debriefing Yoga Practice

Encourage each participant to sit at the front of their mat in a comfortable seated position: "Moving in your own time, find yourself seated at the front of your mat." Then transition into debriefing the practice. Here are some of the questions we often use:

What did you notice?

Did anyone free themselves from the tyranny of their mind, even temporarily?

What gets in the way of that?

What happened next?

Small-Group Exercise: ACT Improv

We get a lot of positive feedback about this exercise. We tell participants that it's like impro-visation in acting and comedy. Improv skits are unscripted. One actor says something, and another actor responds to build on the statement. The actor can't refute what was said but instead must go with it. This process is analogous to psychological flexibility! No matter what thought, feeling, sensation, or memory shows up for us—we go with it.

After offering a brief explanation about what improv is, pass out the ACT Improv work-sheet, which is available for download from this book's website, http://www.newharbinger.com/42358. Have participants break into groups of two. One person from each group should be a sharer, someone who will share a difficult moment from their life, and the other will be the receiver, the person receiving their difficult moment and asking the questions on the worksheet.

Group Dialogue: Debriefing ACT Improv

Invite participants to rejoin the large group and share what they noticed. We generally get positive feedback, such as "That was really amazing," or "It was powerful and so simple." Sometimes we receive seemingly negative feedback, and we troubleshoot in those instances. For example, if someone tells us it felt forced, mechanical, or confining to only ask the questions on the worksheet, we respond with curiosity, trying to clarify what specifically made the improvisation exercise difficult for them.

Oftentimes, we find that people want a lot of backstory, the historical aspects of what the sharer has difficulties with. We validate that this is how the mind can work. It wants more information so it can draw conclusions and come up with explanations. We also offer an explanation of why seeking more information can get the receiver stuck in the details of the story, like getting hooked rather than focusing on learning new ways to relate to that painful content and move forward flexibly.

ACT Improv

Take a breath on purpose. Feel the sensations of breathing. What do you notice right now?

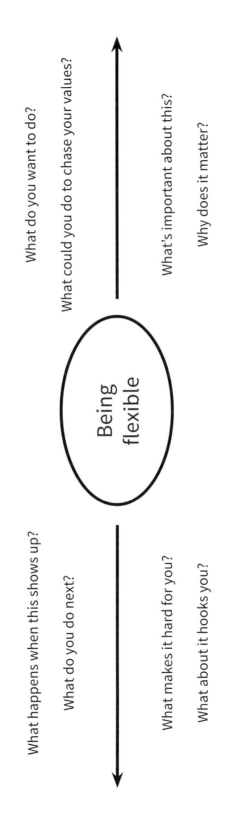

What do you want to do?

What could you do to chase your values?

What's important about this?

Why does it matter?

Being flexible

Where do you feel that in your body?

What thoughts or feelings show up for you?

What happens when this shows up?

What do you do next?

What makes it hard for you?

What about it hooks you?

Session Five Home Practice: Stress Management and Self-Care

Participants may notice that as they attempt to engage in life in a different way that hooks show up in the guise of responsibility, including thoughts like *I don't have time* and feelings of guilt related to being focused on the self rather than on others. For this reason, we focus the at-home practice in session five on stress management and self-care. When we talk about stress management, keep in mind that we're not focusing on trying to control or eliminate stress but on identifying better ways to engage with stress and increase our awareness of our values so we can live a more meaningful life.

Have participants work in pairs to complete the Connect with You: Self-Care Life Map, which is available for download at this book's website, http://www.newharbinger.com /42358. Using this worksheet, participants will identify ways to take care of themselves that are meaningful to them, private experiences, stressors that show up and get in the way of self-care, what they do when these impediments show up (usually choosing not to do the self-care activity), and what specific self-care behaviors are consistent with their values. The end goal is for them to derive at least one daily self-care practice, such as taking five minutes to write in a gratitude journal every morning or completing a stretching routine every evening before bed, and three self-care behaviors that they can do that take less than ten minutes each. The hope is that participants can develop a regular self-care practice and also identify a couple of extra self-care behaviors they can incorporate into days when needed. They will write these down in the top-right quadrant, where their commitments go.

Connect with You: Self-Care Life Map

Part 1. Provide at least one answer in each quadrant.

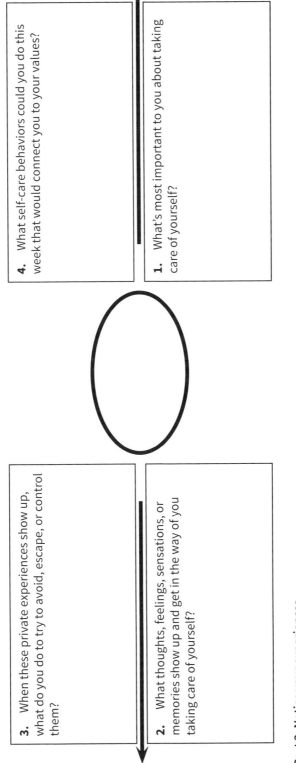

4. What self-care behaviors could you do this week that would connect you to your values?

1. What's most important to you about taking care of yourself?

3. When these private experiences show up, what do you do to try to avoid, escape, or control them?

2. What thoughts, feelings, sensations, or memories show up and get in the way of you taking care of yourself?

Part 2. Notice your experiences.

- What does it feel like to take time for yourself?

- What does it feel like to move away from painful thoughts, feelings, sensations, and memories?

- Do you spend the majority of your life taking care of yourself or trying to avoid painful experiences?

Ending Savasana: Meditation on Sound

For this ending Savasana, you'll need a bell or a smartphone with a bell sound.

In the resting position of Savasana, come back to the simplicity of the breath moving in the body, feeling the breath and also drawing the ear to hear the breath.

For this lying meditation, we'll focus on sound. I'll invite you to open up to the experience of sound and the practice of deep listening.

In a moment, I will ring a bell. Once the bell is rung, do your best to follow the sound of the bell from start to finish.

[*Ring the bell once or twice, allowing the tone to fade completely before ringing it again.*]

As the you hear the bell, use the sound not only as an anchor to hold your attention, but also as something to come back to when the mind wanders.

[*Ring the bell one to three times.*]

Notice how the mind begins to place language on the sound, labels like pretty, calming, terrible, loud…many layers. Just note to yourself that the comments may describe the sound, but they are not the actual experience of sound… Can you go back to the sound?

[*Ring the bell.*]

Allow the sound to simply be. You cannot control the sound. Just let it flow into the ear.

[*Ring the bell.*]

Allow the sound to come to you.

[*Ring the bell one to three times.*]

A microphone does not choose what sounds come in and what sounds do not. It's open to all the sounds that come its way.

[*Ring the bell two to five times.*]

Maintain this practice of deep listening, open to sound without attending to anything specific… When you're ready, start to feel a slightly deeper and longer inhale and exhale.

In your own time, roll onto your right side, using the left hand to raise yourself up. Come to be seated at the front of your mat to begin our good-bye ritual.

Once all participants are seated at the top of their mat, end this fifth session of MYACT as you ended session one, with chanting, sharing appreciations, and a closing posture.

Working with Individuals

- Instead of the self-disclosure card shuffle exercise, you may choose to share something you're struggling with, and how that shows up in the therapy session, and then have the client do the same. For example, being vulnerable is difficult for most people due to past hurts, so the client may make jokes to avoid uncomfortable conversations. You may worry that you aren't doing a good job or feel uncomfortable with conflict, so you may avoid pushing the client to sit with discomfort, or you might not call them out on in-session avoidance behaviors when doing so would benefit them.

- You can use ACT improv (without the worksheet) to talk through a situation or problem you're working on with a client. The improv process also challenges you to be more flexible in how you approach the client's presenting problems.

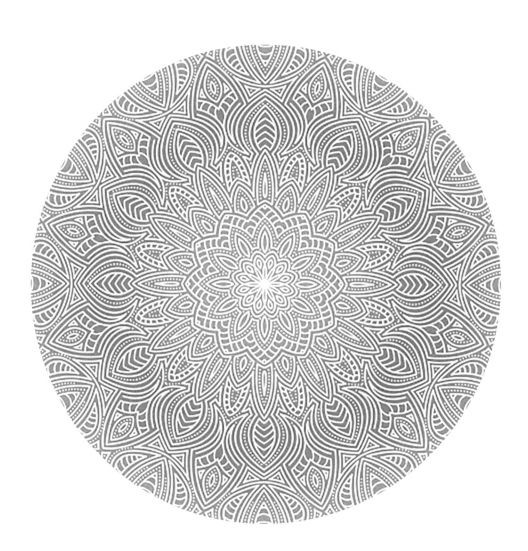

Vipassanā

In yoga, *vipassanā* is the action or technology of living life. Through vipassanā, yoga asks practitioners to see themselves as completely separate from the content of the mind, and from this detached place, to live in congruence with cosmic law. The contextual behavioral science approach of ACT internalizes this difficult perspective and more easily defines vipassanā as seeing the self as the context of what is experienced, not the content, and acknowledging that it's possible to be detached from content. This approach uniquely mediates for positive outcomes. We interpret the cosmic law of yoga as simply meaning to align behaviors with values, the distal reinforcers we karmically established in session four. So in this sixth session of MYACT, we'll bring the spiritual focus of yoga to the forefront using the contextual behavioral science tools of deictic framing (perspective taking).

In this session, you'll specifically build upon the defusion processes from session five, in which participants interacted with their difficult experiences in new ways. The exercises in this session encourage participants to undertake self-as-process and self-as-context experiential work and seek to evoke a spiritual, transcendent sense of self. Depending on your practice setting and cultural context, it may be necessary to explicitly state that the yoga we'll be doing is a nonreligious practice. In the following beginning meditation, we suggest allowing extralong pauses. This additional time allows participants to be in silence, noticing their experience.

Beginning Meditation: You Are Not Your Body

Find yourself in Savasana. Allow yourself to find stillness in your body. Take a breath on purpose. Breathe all the way in. Really feel the air enter your body as the belly expands. Pause and feel the sensations of your body filled with air. Exhale all the way. Feel the belly collapse as air is pushed out of your body.

Allow your breath to return to its normal pace. Notice that your body continues to work at breathing, drawing oxygen in on the inhale and pushing air out on the exhale. This process of breathing continues without your conscious effort. Just as you are not the air that you breathe in, that you are separate from the circulatory system that draws in oxygen and gives nutrients to your blood, know that the you that is hearing my voice and noticing your breath is separate from the sound of my voice. You are not my voice and you are not the sensations of your breath. You are no more one with your body than you are one with the trees that photosynthesize oxygen. You are aware of all these varied experiences, but you are not these experiences.

Group Dialogue: Debriefing Home Practice

Encourage participants to reflect on their MYACT practice over the past week. The debriefing is an opportunity to talk about how the home practice went for participants, to reinforce their engagement in new behaviors, and also to troubleshoot problems that may have arisen. Here are some prompts you can use to get the discussion going:

Before we move on, how did everyone feel after they went home last week?

Did you have any difficulty or success completing the Connect with You: Self-Care Life Map worksheet?

How was it to do this practice?

What did you notice while doing it?

Did any hooks show up around actually completing the Connect with You: Self-Care Life Map worksheet?

Did you commit yourself to any values-based action this week related to taking care of yourself?

Your Two Futures

This perspective-taking meditation offers participants the opportunity to view two different futures: one in which nothing changes and one in which they move toward their values. It provides them an opportunity to bring distal (long-term) outcomes into the present moment to encourage change.

Allowing your eyes to close, or keeping them open and dropping the gaze or softening the focus, take a breath on purpose. Really take care of yourself in this moment. Maybe bring some motion into your body. Do whatever you need to do to be successful and engaged with this meditation. Really use flexibility here to choose what's right for you.

With the idea of health in mind as a value, whatever that means to you—physical, emotional, spiritual health—connect with what is meaningful to you about engaging in health-related behaviors, whatever that looks like in your life. Take stock of how you're living your life right now, noticing if you're moving toward a life that's meaningful to you, noticing areas of strength, and also noticing areas that ask for improvement. Receiving a clear picture of how you live your life from day to day and how that relates to your values.

For example, I'm imagining coming home from work at eight o'clock and immediately putting on my pajamas, sitting in this big chair I have, and relaxing instead of going to the gym, like I told myself I would. This is a simple act of me taking care of myself.

As you are thinking about what you might be doing in your current life, I want you to fast-forward ten years into the future. If there are events that happened in the ten years, allow your mind to stop on those moments, but imagine yourself ten years from now and what your life would look like if you changed nothing in how you're living your life. Imagine all the behaviors you're doing or not doing just stayed the same. Pause and ask yourself where you'd be in ten years. Not thinking abstractly, but looking in the mirror of your ten-years-older self, what do you look like? Are you working? Who's in your life? What are you spending your free time doing? Really getting a clear picture of what your life looks like.

Then noticing if you feel like you're walking in the direction of those values in this ten-years-older version of yourself. Maybe you're still in the same spot you're in now. Paying attention to how that feels. Are you where you want to be ten years from now, if nothing changed? Really be curious about any reaction you have.

As we pull back to this moment, hold on to the image of yourself, your life, and its details, particularly the emotional details. If your eyes are closed, gently opening your eyes, jotting down a few things about what stuck out most to you. Write just a couple of things to jog your memory, even bullet points.

Then going back, if you're willing, to an eyes-closed posture, or allowing your vision to soften. I want you to think back to your life map and all the behaviors in the top-right quadrant that represent your value of whole health. Imagining your life right now, envision yourself every day incorporating one of those things into your life. What if every day you paused and asked yourself, What is one step I could take to move toward a value of health, playfulness, adventure, connection, self-care?

If you could take one step every day toward that value, imagine yourself ten years from now. Looking at yourself in the mirror, what do you look like? Working, not working? What are you spending your free time doing? Just allow that image to permeate your consciousness and realize that I'm not suggesting you wonder what life would be like if you were perfect. This isn't the most perfect time line, the one in which you make all your New Year's resolutions, you are a fitness goddess or god, you always follow through on plans, and you have grand adventures. For example, small behaviors I might do to move toward a value include standing up and dancing, taking a brief walk, and doing one pull-up. Where would you be ten years from now?

Again, as we pull ourselves back into the present moment, bring with you a snapshot of your life, not just what you're doing and what you look like but what it feels like to move in the direction of taking daily steps toward your values. Again, if your eyes are closed, opening your eyes and writing down things that you noticed that stuck out to you.

Whoever feels comfortable sharing that experience, I'd like to invite you to do so.

Group Dialogue: Debriefing Your Two Futures

Take some time to poll the group about their experience of the your two futures meditation. What stood out to them? Were the two futures very different or similar? What images came to mind? Ask if anyone would feel comfortable sharing the notes they jotted down about each future. Really connect them with the idea that neither future is right or wrong, but rather each is an opportunity to investigate the outcomes of the path they're on now and of the work we're doing in these sessions.

Yoga Is Self-Compassion

In this session, so far we've been using deictic framing to help participants separate the seer from the content of the mind. Having distance from this content can be a feat in and of itself. Practicing being kind to the self is even more challenging, especially considering the Western cultural implications of being outcome focused, a perspective that now dominates much of the globe. The yogic practice shifts one's perspective from self-as-content to self-as-process in order to achieve the perspective of self-as-context, meaning the seer views the self as the context of all experience. This is easier said than done, which is why we included specific yoga cues to free participants from self-conceptualizations. These cues encourage participants to flexibly adapt to the challenges that arise physically in the asanas and prāṇāyāma, or breath work.

For example, during a physically challenging posture, you can encourage participants to use the breath as a tool of attention, listening to how and where they feel its movements in order to inform what they might do next: go deeper into a posture, back out a little, back out a lot, or perhaps take a break. Or by being reminded to practice noticing, participants may realize they are holding their breath in a particularly difficult posture. This may lead them to turn more attention to that area to soften it and draw the breath into it, or to notice thoughts, feelings, or sensations that arise during this posture. From the perspective of the seer, we can observe the world and the way we interact with it, ultimately showing ourselves kindness in the process.

Before starting the yoga practice, introduce the idea of the seer:

There is a you there behind your eyes. It was the same you who prepared to come here for this session, the same you who was there behind your eyes at our first session. Do you remember that? Imagine your body is a vessel and that your true self is looking out through your eyes as if they're portholes. We've been focusing on this concept throughout this session. Having you look from different perspectives—at two different futures, at yourself in different situations—is all about recognizing that you are separate from what you experience. This is your true self, and by settling into your natural state, you're free to choose how you behave and how you interact with yourself. It can be so easy for us to beat up on ourselves when we face difficulty. In this yoga practice, you're going to face suffering, and I'm going to ask you to meet it from the distance of your true self, to be with your judgments, evaluations, and difficult sensations, and to engage with yourself lovingly. I'm going to ask you to give yourself the nurturance you need to thrive.

After the introduction, conduct the sixth yoga sequence, comprising the following practices:

- Standing Half-Sun Salutations (continuous)

- Chaturanga Push-Ups

- Locust

- Downward Dog

- Locust to Downward Dog (transition)

- Boat

- Supported Lying Twists

- Leg Up the Wall

To start, lead the group through continuous **Standing Half-Sun Salutations**, as described in session five. From there, you'll move into strengthening postures, a focus of this session's yoga practice.

There is this notion that yoga is all about being flexible and bendy and putting your body into impressive shapes. And although mobility is important for functional living, it's essential that we also have enough strength and stability to support a range of motion. The following postures focus on building strength and stability in the hips, legs, shoulders, arms, and core.

Chaturanga Push-Ups

Chaturanga Push-Ups are slightly different than the regular push-up most of us are familiar with. Whereas a regular push-up has a wide hand position, with the elbows out away from the rib cage, while performing a Chaturanga Push-Up, the hands are shoulder-width apart, with the elbows closer to the ribs. In the world of strength and conditioning, this movement is known as a triceps push-up.

To start, come into Table. From there, walk the hands slightly forward so the thighs and pelvis move closer to the floor. With the shoulders over the wrists, the torso, hips, and thighs will be in one straight line [low plank]. The creases on top of the wrists will be relatively parallel to the front of your mat, and your middle fingers should face straight forward. A modification is to have the fingers angle slightly out to the side [external rotation of the shoulder]. This allows the wrists and shoulders of some to find a more manageable position. If the wrists feel painful and compressed, you can do this movement on fists so the wrists stay neutral.

Actively but not aggressively, press the hands into the mat. As you do that, feel how the shoulder blades move away from the spine a little. This helps the shoulders to be more stable as you lower down.

To begin the movement, keep rooting down from the shoulders into the hands as you begin to bend the elbows [shoulder extension and elbow flexion]. As you lower yourself, the upper arms will find a position relatively parallel to the rib cage and the chest will move closer to the floor. As the shoulders and elbows move, the hips and thighs will also move closer to the floor. As you slowly lower down, try to notice if at any point in the movement you feel the shoulders begin to round forward, the collarbones narrow, or the shoulder blades begin to lift toward the ears [elevation]. These are all signs of compensation. You want the shoulder blades to remain stable and the collarbones to remain broad, so only go as close to the floor as you can while maintaining this posture.

As you practice this movement to the level that allows you to keep proper form, more depth will become available as you get stronger and more stable. From your appropriate depth, press yourself back up to the starting position without locking the elbows.

We recommend five to fifteen repetitions, depending on the strength and stamina of each individual and the context of the particular session. As the body fatigues through the movement, it's okay to decrease the range of motion within the movement to suit the amount of strength available. Chaturanga Push-Ups can also be done against a wall, a countertop, or a table. This alternative is especially good for participants who have difficulty lowering down to and rising from the floor. As participants gain more strength and stability through practice, it might become an option to do Chaturanga Push-Ups with the knees raised off the floor, keeping in mind that this variation requires more strength.

We can't stress enough that our approach to movement is not about the "final goal." It's not about being able to bang out fifteen rounds of Chaturanga Push-Ups or holding a difficult position for a really long period of time. Our approach is more about the movement serving as a tool to practice mindfulness. For sure, increased strength, stamina, and mobility are fantastic potential by-products of practicing these postures and movements, just like calmness is a wonderful potential by-product of meditation practice. But they're not the goal.

Locust (Prone Backbend)

To begin Locust, lie on your mat with the belly resting on the floor, arms at your sides, legs straight, toes pointed back, and head turned to one side. Pause here for a few breaths, connecting to the sensations of breath moving through the body. Remember that when we talk about yoga as a tool for practicing mindfulness, this really means practicing feeling. Yoga is a tool for practicing feeling the experience of breathing; for practicing feeling the movements happening in the body; for practicing feeling how the body and breath respond to the movements and postures; as well as for noticing the kinds of things that arise internally for us as we practice feeling these things. As we practice, we connect to what's really happening in the moment.

From this prone, lying position, begin to press down lightly through the tops of the toes. When you do this correctly, you should feel your kneecaps lift slightly away from the mat. If you have a tendency to hyperextend, or lock out, the knees, press down into the floor with less force so you don't hyperextend. Brace the abdomen; contract as if you're about to get poked in the stomach.

Actively but not aggressively, draw the shoulder blades in toward the spine and down away from the ears. This first movement [retraction] will broaden the chest and lift the collarbones away from the floor. A good way to visualize the movement is to imagine that you're squeezing a pencil between the shoulder blades. On an inhale, start to lift the chest away from the floor by contracting the muscles along your spine [spinal extension]. As you lift up, the arms will also lift away from the floor and up toward the ceiling.

If while you're in the position you notice discomfort arising along the spine, decrease the amount of effort you're putting into the lift. Remember, we're interested in quality of movement, not quantity.

You can hold Locust anywhere from three to ten breaths. A common variation for this posture is to lightly squeeze the glutes, which can decrease the tendency to overextend in the low spine. Another option is to take a thinly rolled-up towel or blanket and place it across the low belly to help the pelvis tilt back (posterior tilt), which decreases any hyperextension of the low spine.

Downward Dog

Start in Table. As you press from the shoulders down into the hands, feel a broadness across the upper back as the shoulder blades move slightly away from the spine. Begin to lift the knees away from the floor, taking the hips up and back, while keeping the spine neutral. As you lift the hips and back, the upper arms will fall more in line with the ears; however, depending on the function of the shoulders, the arms and ears may not be perfectly in line.

You can slowly straighten the legs, but if you notice that the spine begins to round out or the shoulders start to shift back over the wrists, keep the knees bent. There is a common misconception that the legs have to be straight in Downward Dog and the feet flat on the floor. This is not true. Straight legs and heels moving toward the floor might eventually become available to you, depending on how the body responds to the position over time. As the hips and shoulders move you into the posture, it's important for the spine to remain neutral and for the breath to maintain its smooth quality, so only straighten the knees to the point that this stays true for you. If while holding the posture the shoulders and neck start to feel irritated, try taking the hands wider than shoulder width. Another good option is to allow the fingers to angle out slightly while adding gentle external rotation to the upper arms.

If on any given day the body is not feeling strong or perhaps you're working with a shoulder, elbow, or wrist injury, it might not be appropriate to do Downward Dog with the knees off the floor. Puppy Dog might be a better option. For this pose, come back to Table and walk the legs and hips back without moving the hands. As the hips shift back, the spine stays long and the upper arms move closer to the side of the skull (flexion). Participants should move back only as far as feels appropriate for the shoulders. With Puppy Dog, we can still work on spinal length and hip and shoulder stability and mobility without forcing all of the body weight into the position.

Locust to Downward Dog (Transition)

It's good to point out to participants that this transition can be extremely difficult for some. It's a movement that takes practice to execute well. Part of the reason for the challenging nature of the transition is neuromuscular. This transition involves movement that we don't often do in daily life, and for that reason, participants' coordination can be shaky and disjointed at first. We like to tell participants to go slowly with this one, and to take their time. The Chaturanga Push-Up, done well, helps with the transition. Through movement, this push-up teaches us to recognize what a strong and solid core feels like.

To start, once you've lifted up into Locust, allow the body to lower down out of the backbend. Place the hands, palms facing down, beside the chest. Have a little spread through the fingers. Keeping the knees on the floor, press down from the shoulders into the hands, and on an exhale, press yourself back up to a low plank, the same starting position for the Chaturanga Push-Up.

Just like when we do the push-up, we're trying to keep a straight line from the knees to the head as we come up from the ground. The movement might be a little bit floppy at first while you're working on coordination and stability.

Once you've pushed up to low plank, make sure your toes are tucked under. Exhale as you begin to lift the hips up and back, hinging at the hip crease and coming into Downward Dog as the upper arms move to more of an overhead position. Remember as you move into Downward Dog to only straighten the legs to the point at which the spine can remain neutral.

From Downward Dog, inhale to come forward into a low plank. On an exhale, lower down through the Chaturanga Push-Up. Sometimes this is not an easy place to hang out, so there is the option to hold a low plank. This pausing in a plank not only allows you to work on the stability of the position, it also helps you to practice slowing down to check the quality of your attention before you lower through the Chaturanga Push-Up. [As we say in classes all the time, "It's not about speeding up to get through it. It's about slowing down to get into it." A very Tantrik perspective.]

Once down, belly on the floor, inhale to Locust. Exhale to lower down. Pause for an inhale to set up the hands. Exhale to press up to plank. Pause for an inhale and then exhale back to Downward Dog.

You can do this sequence from two to ten times, depending on the strength, stability, and stamina of participants in any given session. As we recommended above for the transition from plank to the Chaturanga Push-Up, you could pause participants between each movement. In session seven, we add this sequence to Standing Half-Sun Salutations to make them Standing Full-Sun Salutations.

Boat

Start seated with your knees bent and feet flat on the floor. Take a hold of the backs of the legs for assistance at first. Rooting down into the mat through the sit bones, roll the pelvis slightly forward. Lengthen up through spine, drawing the shoulder blades softly toward the spine, and lightly reach up through the crown of the head. As you add effort to sit up a little taller, make sure the upper shoulders and neck can be soft. Alternatively, sitting on a block to elevate the pelvis or having the feet farther from hips can help you find ease even within the effort, especially if the front of hips or low spine are feeling achy.

From the seated upright position, without rounding the spine, hinge from the hips to lean the torso back. As you lean back, feel how the abdomen becomes more active. This is the core engaging. The objective with Boat is not to lean back as far as you can but instead to lean back to the point where the core becomes active in order to support the spine, the breath can remain smooth, and the hips or low back, or both, do not get irritated. Again, using a little bit of arm strength in this position is fine.

As a way to challenge the body more, when it's appropriate, here are some variations we like to provide as options to participants. They are listed from easiest to hardest:

- Lift one foot off the floor and then the other in an alternating pattern.

- Lift both feet off the floor at the same time.

- Raise your shins to be more parallel with the mat when the legs are off the floor.

- Straighten the legs only to the point before the spine starts to excessively round out (flexion).

- Decrease the effort in the arms, maybe even removing the hands from the legs.

These options are by no means simply a checklist to move through so that you can get to the "end." Ideally, the variation of Boat we choose is appropriate for the level of strength and stamina within any given session. That means that some days the legs may be straight, with no hands, and some days might require feet on the floor and hands on the legs. Try to meet the body where it is instead of trying to make it something different than what it is. Some days we might start in a position that requires more strength and then transition to easier positions as the body fatigues. This is a wonderful way of practicing adapting to what's arising in the present moment (functional contextualism), which really is the practice of upāya (skillful means).

After participants have finished Boat, have them lie on their back and complete a series of **Supported Lying Twists**, as described in session one, and then **Legs Up the Wall**, as described in session three, to finish out this round of yoga.

Group Dialogue: Debriefing Yoga Practice

Encourage participants to sit at the front of their yoga mats in a seated posture that is comfortable for them: "Moving in your own time, find yourself seated at the front of your mat." Debrief the practice with a few questions, such as these:

What did you notice in that practice?

What was it like to move your body in ways that you may not normally move in your everyday life?

Did you get hooked?

Did you find yourself wanting to speed through the postures or try to push yourself into a position your body was not ready for?

Connecting to Your Future Self

This exercise builds upon the perspective taking we've used in previous MYACT sessions. The worksheet participants will work with has them focus explicitly on new behaviors in the presence of a painful situation in the future. This sixth session, including this exercise, is meant to underpin the practice of self-compassion, covered in session seven. We've found it difficult to effectively train self-compassion practices if participants don't have a strong experiential grasp of perspective taking and acceptance processes. Pass out Connecting to Your Future Self worksheets to each participant and have them break into pairs. As done in prior exercises, one person in the pair will ask the other person the questions found on the worksheet, writing in their answers, then they'll switch roles. You can download the worksheet, along with other accessories for this book, at http://www.newharbinger.com/42358.

Connecting to Your Future Self

This exercise is about picturing yourself in a future situation that could be difficult for you. You may wish to write your responses to each question below. Do your best to really picture yourself in that future situation and to communicate with that future version of yourself.

1. Your future
    - Call to mind a painful situation you anticipate having to face…

    _____

    _____

2. Being there, now
    - What would you see or hear? Can you envision yourself there?

    _____

    _____

3. Speak
    - Can you here, now, in this moment speak to your future self who's in pain?
    - What words or gestures can you share with your future self?

    _____

    _____

4. Receive
    - How does the future version of yourself receive those words or gestures?

    _____

    _____

5. Your needs
    - What tone of voice or posture do you use with this future version of yourself?
    - What might you need in that future situation, when you're in pain?

    _____

    _____

6. Validate
    - Share from your heart, here, now, that you know it's hard, maybe really hard, for that version of your future self.

    _____

    _____

Group Dialogue: Debriefing Connecting to Your Future Self

Take some time to check in with participants about their experience of the Connecting to Your Future Self exercise. If after receiving some feedback, participants haven't naturally begun to share specific details about the content of the exercise, we recommend probing deeper: "Could you see your future self in a difficult situation? What happened when you interacted with that version of you?"

Session Six Home Practice: Healthy Relationships

One way we can learn to take perspective is to try to see the world from behind the eyes of someone we love, which is part of what this session's home practice is about. Each participant will choose a person with whom they are in a relationship (partner, friend, parent, child), and then each of them will complete the Working Together: Relationship Life Map worksheet (available for download at http://www.newharbinger.com/42358) to identify the values that underlie the relationship and the hooks that show up and get in the way of them being their best in the relationship. After completing the top portion of the worksheet on their own, the two will come together to share their experiences and create a workable plan for moving forward in the relationship.

This exercise offers them an important opportunity to discuss support, both the support of family and friends as well as professional support. Encourage the participants to undertake this discussion with their chosen loved one, so they can identify the supportive people in their lives and the ways that they are supportive of each other. Examples of the latter include being a good listener, creating a safe space for the other to experience unpleasant emotions, and encouraging social interactions by making regular plans with them. Additionally, encourage participants to identify resources in their community that can offer support, including 24-hour crisis lines, therapists in the area who do therapy from an ACT perspective (contextualscience.org has a directory of therapists who self-identify as ACT therapists), any free mental health or wellness resources in the community (such as community centers, peer support groups, community events), and so on. The idea is for them to create a context for support seeking in the home, at work, and in the community, while at the same time working to understand how individual patterns of responding may influence patterns between people.

Working Together: Relationship Life Map

Answer the questions in section 1 individually, and use that information to generate answers to the second section, in which you'll together plan what to do next.

Section 1 (Partner 1)

Why do "we" matter? What about this relationship is important to me?

_____

_____

_____

What do I want to be about in this relationship?

_____

_____

_____

What hooks me?

_____

_____

_____

What do I do when I get hooked?

_____

_____

_____

How do I want to respond when I see a hook?

_____

_____

_____

Section 1 (Partner 2)

Why do "we" matter? What about this relationship is important to me?

_____

_____

_____

What do I want to be about in this relationship?

_____

_____

_____

What hooks me?

_____

_____

_____

What do I do when I get hooked?

_____

_____

_____

How do I want to respond when I see a hook?

_____

_____

_____

Section 2

What do we want to be doing together to move us toward what matters?

_____

_____

_____

_____

_____

_____

_____

What can we do to support one another when we get hooked?

_____

_____

_____

_____

_____

_____

_____

_____

_____

_____

Ending Savasana or Seated Meditation: Seeing the World in New Ways

Find yourself in Savasana or a comfortable seated position. Throughout this practice, we've been learning how to shift our perspective. A powerful and useful way to work on this new skill is to pause and notice the subtle qualities of what this moment affords, which we can easily take for granted. Even now, as you're breathing and hearing the sound of my voice, what experiences go by unnoticed? Pay extra attention to whatever occurs to you; it need not be profound. Remember, this practice is about your journey, your showing up, and even as I say this practice is about you, what occurs to you that you wouldn't normally notice on purpose? What thoughts or judgments fly by under the radar of your consciousness?

Bring to mind someone or something important to you that you'll interact with in the coming days. Really allow yourself to picture yourself there. What goes by unnoticed? What is underappreciated? In the business of living, seeking goals and objectives, working, completing lists, our senses become dull. What has your awareness become insensitive to? The color of someone's eyes that you love? The sound of their voice? The deeply personal history and connection that shapes the choices you make day in and day out?

Once all participants are seated at the top of their mat, end this sixth session of MYACT as you ended session one, with chanting, sharing appreciations, and a closing posture.

Working with Individuals

◉ The your two futures meditation doesn't have to be about the value of health. You can modify it to fit with a specific non-health-related value the client is struggling with.

◉ You may choose to shorten the yoga practice and focus on Locust to the Downward Dog transition as the strengthening postures. Or you could focus on a pose you've done before, such as Standing Half-Sun Salutation, and have the client, if they're willing, guide you both.

◉ Forgo the Connecting to Your Future Self worksheet and make this exercise a conversation. You can tailor the future difficult situation to focus on whatever you and the client are working on in session.

Karuṇā

During the last session, we began to explore compassion. We waited until this second-to-last MYACT session to expand on the topic because, in our experience, it takes time to train participants in self-compassion. It is difficult to do. Also, we've found that participants have an easier time offering compassion and cultivating self-compassion once they have a strong foundation in accepting and perspective taking. We've noted that many participants understandably see self-compassion and self-love as self-indulgent and not practical in the real world, at least in terms of seeing positive outcomes. We also believe participants must meet certain conditions before they can formulate authentic compassion. The practitioner must be physically vital and psychologically flexible; be in contact with their varied experiences of emotions, thoughts, sensations, and memories; and have the ability and desire to act with intention in accordance with their values. At this point in MYACT, participants should be meeting these criteria.

In this session, you'll explore *karuṇā*, the Buddhist and Jain concept of removing suffering and harm from the world. The sages understood that wisdom is wonderful, and that it must be obtained through living: the path must be walked, the world requires doing. To cultivate a deeper understanding of karuṇā, you'll invite participants to let go of struggles with specific content in an acceptance-inspired present-moment meditation, among other exercises. This session has a longer yoga practice that combines many of the previous sessions' skills, creating both a fluid yoga practice and a more challenging setting in which to practice accepting the self.

Beginning Meditation: Right Now, It's Like This

Settling into a relaxed pose that's comfortable for you, take a breath on purpose and notice your experience, whatever shows up for you in this moment: the judgment of the quality of your breath, whether it's shallow or deep, the comfort of settling into a familiar space and practice, the dull ache of the lower back or other pain in the body. Breathe it in to really acknowledge it. Breathe out, saying to yourself, *In this moment, it's like this.*

Inhale to expand your awareness beyond the sensations of settling into this moment, and bring your awareness to the felt, emotional experience of entering this space and beginning this practice. What feelings are coming through the door with you? Perhaps you were feeling rushed or hopeful before entering this space. Take a moment to pause and come in full contact with what it feels like to be here, now. Notice if your mind has an opinion about how you ought to feel or if it keeps trying to pull you somewhere else. And in this moment, acknowledge, *Right now, it's like this.*

Reflect on your time in this space, the work you've done, the new behaviors you've engaged in, the subtle shifts in your perspective. Remember the first day that you began this work, what it was like to be there behind your eyes, what you hoped to get from our time together. Notice that it's the same you, there, behind your eyes, thinking, feeling, sensing, remembering, observing. You have changed, yet it's the same you whose been there this whole time on this journey. As you reflect on your experience of walking this path, notice what it's like to look back and see where you've come from, standing where you are now, and, even now, simply reaffirm: *Right now, it's like this.*

As we prepare ourselves for this session and the work that we'll do together, give yourself permission to be fully in contact with what the moment affords you. Allow yourself to restate, *Right now, it's like this.*

Group Dialogue: Debriefing Home Practice

Encourage participants to reflect on their MYACT practice over the past week. The debriefing of the home practice is an opportunity to talk about how home practice went for participants, to reinforce their engagement in new behaviors, and also to troubleshoot problems that may have arisen. We've found these prompts helpful for stimulating the conversation:

Before we move on, how did everyone feel after they went home last week?

Did you have any difficulty or success completing the Working Together: Relationship Life Map worksheets?

How was it to do this practice?

What did you notice while doing it?

Did you commit yourself to any values-based action this week related to improving your meaningful relationship?

How did it go?

Placard Moments

For this exercise, hand out a sheet of paper and a marker to each participant. Make sure participants are aware of what will happen in this activity before they consent to participate. Explain that they'll be invited to write something important on the sheet and then show it to other members in the group. Remind participants that if they wish to not write or share, they can still participate by observing the group interaction. Instruct them to write large enough so that if they were to hold up their sheet like a placard, someone standing across from them could read it clearly. Then you'll describe what to write on the placard and how the exercise works.

> Take a moment to pause and reflect on something that's important to you in life. It could be a difficult situation you're dealing with or something that you're particularly proud of. Whatever shows up in your heart, connect with it for a moment and see if you can articulate it in writing on your placard. Your description needn't be long or include a lot of details. Write down just what's important—what is in your heart.
>
> [We give participants two to four minutes to complete their placards, and upon completion, we collect the markers and tell them that this exercise will be a sort of walking meditation.] In this exercise, I'm inviting you to walk around the room in silence, to greet each other with your eyes, and then to hold up your placard for the other to read. Read each placard, and pause for a moment to connect in a way that feels safe and respectful before continuing to walk. You may stop and pause, sharing a moment with the same person more than once. You may wish to sit down and take time to yourself during the exercise. When the music ends, please find yourself seated back at your yoga mat, again in silence. We'll take some time to debrief the exercise and make sense of what we experienced.

We ring a bell to mark the beginning of the exercise and play "Lent et Douloureux" from Erik Satie's *Gymnopédies*. We find this score appropriate, as it is an atmospheric, minimalist piece with major and minor movements that elicit a variety of moods.

Yoga Is Practice

Before starting this session's yoga practice, facilitate a brief discussion about how important being engaged with one's life is. We try to be as reinforcing as possible, explaining that showing up to this group, taking the time to confront one's painful history, might be acts of chasing one's values. In our experience, taking some time to reflect on earlier MYACT sessions, describing seemingly innocuous behaviors that participants did in the context of the group that were viewed as improvements in behavior, is helpful. Perhaps someone said something particularly vulnerable, or another participant took a risk in the group. Whatever example you choose, emphasize the doing: how the particular participant exemplified the qualities of chasing something meaningful. We transition out of this discussion by saying, "This week's yoga practice is about the same thing: behaving in a way that is in line with your values, walking the path of what matters to you."

In yoga asana practice, it's common to hear instructors say, "Yoga is not about the poses." The forms, the movements, the breathing are all a context for practicing attention. It is through the body and mind that we move through this life. Another phrase you might also hear, which we're not fans of, is "full expression," as in "Move toward the full expression," or "If the full expression of the posture isn't available, do this modification." "Full expression" has the potential to create the idea that participants are not where they're supposed to be and that they should work really hard to get to that dreamlike posture. Once there they'll feel complete and "full." From a Tantrik perspective, this couldn't be further from the truth.

Within this protocol, we encourage participants to work from where they are, not where they think they're supposed to be. In this regard, the destination we're trying to get to is right here. Therefore, the "full expression" of any pose is based on what is available to us in any given moment. This is clearly highlighted with a phrase that often gets passed around yoga teacher trainings and throughout yoga studies: "We don't use our body to get into these poses; we use the poses to get into our body" (Clark, 2012, 23). We go even go further by saying, "We use the poses to get into our life."

You'll now conduct the seventh yoga sequence, comprising the following practices:

- Standing Half-Sun Salutations (continuous)

- Standing Full-Sun Salutations

- Supported Lying Twists

- Legs Up the Wall

To start the active practice, lead the group through continuous **Standing Half-Sun Salutations**, as described in session five.

Standing Full-Sun Salutations

To begin, stand at the front of your mat with the feet at hip width. Connecting to the feeling of your breath moving in and moving out, inhale to reach the arms up toward the ceiling. As you reach up, there is also the option to take your gaze toward the hands, but if this irritates the neck, feel free to keep the neck neutral and relaxed.

As you exhale, tilt the pelvis forward as you move into Standing Forward Fold. As the body folds forward, try to feel that the movement starts at the pelvis so that you are not just rounding your spine. Ideally, the spine stays long as you fold until the pelvis can't tilt forward anymore, at which point the spine begins to round. As you're coming into your Standing Forward Fold, it's also important to not lock your knees. They should remain slightly bent. When you find your Standing Forward Fold, have enough bend in the knees so that the low belly can rest on the upper thighs.

From there, keeping the knees bent, place your hands on your shins. As you inhale, contract the muscles in the back to lift and lengthen your spine. As you lengthen the spine, draw the shoulder blades together toward the midline. On a slow exhale, release the hands to the mat and take the legs back one at a time to find your plank. Take a breath or two here to set up the arms for Chaturanga Push-Ups and to decide whether it's appropriate to do the push-ups on your knees or toes. Remember that doing them on your toes isn't necessarily better than your knees, it's just harder.

On an exhale, lower down through Chaturanga. As you come down to the belly and chest, keep the breath moving as you point through the toes and bring the arms to your sides. On an inhale, lift up into Locust. Exhale to lower down. Stay attentive to the breath as you bring the hands into position to press back up to plank.

On your next exhale, rooting down from the shoulders into the hands, press up to plank. With toes tucked under, lift the hips up and back to Downward Dog or Puppy Dog, depending on how strong you feel. And hold as long as feels appropriate.

With a slow exhale, step toward the hands, finding your Standing Forward Fold. As you inhale, allow the spine to round toward the legs. Exhale to pause and sink into your fold. As you inhale, return to a standing position as you lift the arms up overhead. Exhale to bring the hands to heart center.

Inhale to Standing Forward Fold, and exhale to place your hands on your shins. As you inhale, contract through the muscles in the back to lift and lengthen your spine. Exhale into your Standing Forward Fold. Inhale as you rise back to standing, reaching the arms up overhead. Exhale, bringing the hands to heart center. Take a moment to consciously attend to what might be arising—sensations, breathing, sounds, thinking.

[We recommend doing this sequence one to five times. Remind participants that the more rounds they do, the more they might fatigue, and that it's okay to modify a movement or back up, slow down, and take few breaths before continuing to move, if they need to.]

Remember that as you become fatigued, the breath and body will try and communicate that to you. Listening to this feedback is a wonderful opportunity to deepen the connection between mind and body. Listening is one way that we can practice tuning in deeply to the present moment, feeling how the body responds, not in language but in sensations that only we have access to from our unique perspective. Noticing the thoughts that arise out of an experience can offer clarity about the options we have for responding in the moments to follow.

After finishing this series of Standing Full-Sun Salutations, take participants through a series of **Supported Lying Twists**, as described in session one, and then end with **Legs Up the Wall**, as described in session three.

Group Dialogue: Debriefing Yoga Practice

Encourage participants to sit at the front of their yoga mats in a seated posture that's comfortable for them: "Moving in your own time, find yourself seated at the front of your mat." You may want to transition into the debriefing using one or all of the following prompts:

What did you notice in that practice?

What was it like to practice a repetitive movement?

Were you able to notice the changes in your body with each Standing Full-Sun Salutation?

Did any hooks show up for you?

Zen Death Poem Authorship

In this exercise, you'll invite each participant to write a poem. Explain that they'll have time in group to write the poem, but that they may wish to edit or rewrite it between sessions. Be sure to also tell them that everyone will read their poem aloud in the final session of MYACT. Then introduce the concept of the Zen death poem to the group with the following script, or a variation of it.

> In Zen, authoring a small piece of poetry in the spirit of acknowledging and making peace with death is a traditional writing practice. The death poem is about presence in the process of dying. It challenges us to maintain connection with the process of letting go and dying, encouraging us to stay present, to be aware of our experiences, and to reflect on our values.
>
> This little exercise is also about rejoicing. Every year that we're still here to enjoy this life, we celebrate with what we might also call a "just in case" poem on our birthday. This death poem is a celebration of another year but also a recognition of the impermanence of things and of the importance of being present to the unfolding of life and living. Writing this poem is not about being poetic or writing something deeply profound. It's about being explicit about the process of our life, what it means to be alive thus far, and the process of letting things go.

Then explain the structure of the poem. You may want to hand out a printed copy of the poem structure or write it down somewhere everyone can see it:

Line 1: How you see your life in this moment

Line 2: How long you have lived

Line 3: What feelings you have approaching death

Line 4: Your understanding of Zen (life)

After explaining the structure of the poem, but before transitioning into having participants begin writing their death poem, read aloud a personal example, as this helps set the right tone for spending a few minutes writing in silence. Here's an example:

Trying and not trying to be so
many things and nothing,
for thirty-six years, I say I'm not
attached but so much to lose,
cleaning up cat shit, washing dishes,
changing diapers, kissing my wife, this is it.

Group Dialogue: Debriefing Zen Death Poem Authorship

Ring a bell three times to signal the completion of the activity, and then instruct participants to set their paper and writing instruments aside and engage in a debriefing: "In a word or two, let's each take a moment to share how we're feeling in this moment." Go around the circle, with each participant sharing, and then ask, "Would anyone be willing to share their experience of writing their death poem?"

Session Seven Home Practice: Sleep Hygiene

Sleep deficits can be a large barrier to engaging in a meaningful life. After all, when we're tired, it's a lot harder to pay attention and a lot easier to be overwhelmed with irritation, anxiety, and sadness. Review the following sleep hygiene information with participants, asking them questions along the way.

> We're going to discuss strategies for increasing the quality and quantity of sleep. Please answer out loud as I read the questions and pay attention to the information provided. We'll discuss each strategy briefly as we go through the questions. The information may offer you ways to modify your sleep environment, your schedule, and the factors that influence your sleep.

1. Select a standard bedtime and wake-up time.

   Do you fall asleep at the same time every night?

   Do you wake up at the same time every morning?

2. Use the bed only for sleeping.

   Do you read in bed?

   Do you use your phone, tablet, or laptop in bed?

   Do you watch television in bed?

   Do you eat in bed?

3. Get up when you can't sleep.

   Do you get out of bed when you can't sleep?

4. Set environmental factors in your favor.

    Do you watch television before going to bed?

    Is your bedroom dark, quiet, and cool?

5. Cut the caffeine and other stimulants.

    Do you drink caffeine (coffee, soda, tea, energy drinks, and so forth) within six hours of going to bed?

    Do you smoke cigarettes?

6. Avoid alcohol.

    Do you drink alcohol in the evenings, even one glass of wine?

7. Stand up and move.

    Do you exercise for at least ten minutes every day?

Above all, be patient! Sleep problems, like anything else, developed over time, so it will take some time to return to a more normal sleep pattern. After you've gone through this material, ask participants to identify one change they can make in their sleep hygiene that they're willing to try over the next week. Then hand out the Sleep Tracker worksheets (available in downloadable form at http://www.newharbinger.com/42358) for them to use to track their sleep for seven days. We're operating under the assumption that everyone can improve their sleep. If people are sleeping well, ask them to track their patterns and identify

Sleep Tracker

Week: _____

Complete this side *before* going to sleep.

A blue screen is any device that emits blue light (television, laptop, computer, tablet, smartphone, e-reader, and so on) and doesn't shift to warm hues (for example, have an "evening mode" setting).

In the blank box, write in anything you believe may be contributing to your sleep problems that you would like to track, such as medication or the use of a CPAP machine.

Date					
Cups of Caffeine					
Minutes Exercised					
Minutes Napped					
Number of Alcoholic Drinks					
Blue Screen 30 Mins. Before Bed: Yes/No					

Sleep Tracker

Week: _____

Complete this side *upon waking up.*

Please provide estimates for the time rather than looking at the clock at night.

Record what time you first went to bed, what time you fell asleep, the number of times you woke up (not counting the final time you awoke), the number of times you were awake (for more than a few minutes) during the night after initially falling asleep, the last time you woke up, and the time you got out of bed, as well as any comments or observations.

Date						
Time Went to Bed						
Time Actually Fell Asleep						
Number of Times Woke Up						
Total Amount of Time Awake						
Time Last Woke Up						
Time Got Out of Bed						

what they're doing that works. Remind them that sleep is just one more way that we can be kind to ourselves.

Ending Savasana: Self-Compassion

In this session, the closing resting posture includes a story about self-compassion. You can use the one we included or feel free to replace it with another that inspires you or that you think will inspire participants. The story should direct participants to contemplate the ways that they can practice self-compassion or help them recognize the ways they already practice self-compassion that they might not have considered, or both. Have participants lie on their mat in a comfortable position.

> As you rest here, allow your attention to settle on breathing. This final meditation will unfold as a story of a man who met some unexpected challenges at a meditation retreat. As I tell you the story, do your best simply to listen, but also notice what kinds of feelings and thoughts arise around the story. Notice without getting pulled in by them. If you notice yourself getting wrapped up in thinking, just come back to listening.
>
> There once was a man who attended a meditation retreat. This wasn't a simple weekend practice or even a more challenging ten-day silent meditation experience, but rather a thirty-day retreat. The man was motivated to attend at the beginning, excited even, but about a week into the retreat, he started to get sick. He felt so ill that he began to wonder if he should leave the retreat altogether.
>
> Conflicted, he went to see his teacher and told him how sick he was feeling. He explained that he didn't think he could make it through the retreat, and he didn't want to waste his or anyone else's time. He especially didn't want to be a burden, needing someone to take care of him.
>
> The teacher asked if he thought he would be able to stay at the retreat and still take care of himself in the ways that he needed to.
>
> The man replied honestly that he didn't know.
>
> His teacher asked him to sleep on it and make a decision in the morning. After a night of sickness and contemplation, the man spoke to his teacher and decided to continue the retreat.
>
> And he did. He stayed for the entire thirty days.

The teacher reached out to the man at the end of the retreat to see if the man was right, if he had been able to care for himself in the ways he needed. The man exclaimed that he was so happy he'd stayed—that while he hadn't wanted to get sick during the retreat, that even in the midst of being sick, there had been something to learn, something important and precious that needed to be taken care of.

In the contemplative traditions, it's common for practitioners to question if they can take care of this moment. Can I meet what is arising without immediately trying to push it away or change it? Can I hold this moment as it is?

Spend a moment here in contemplation. What do you have to take care of? How do you take care of yourself? How could you take care of yourself?

In time, add some depth to your inhales and length to your exhales. Layer on whatever movements seem necessary.

In your own time, roll onto your right side, using the left hand to raise yourself up. Come to be seated at the front of your mat to begin our ritual of saying good-bye.

Once all participants are seated at the top of their mat, end this seventh session of MYACT as you ended session one, with chanting, sharing appreciations, and a closing posture.

Working with Individuals

- For the placard moments exercise, you may choose to have the client write something on a card and read it to you or have a discussion about what they chose to share, or both. Individual sessions often create a space in which clients focus on painful or difficult situations in life, so reflecting on something that's important to them may be a new experience. Though clients may struggle to identify meaningful moments when first meeting with you, by this point in the protocol, they should have something meaningful to connect with. This exercise can offer them the opportunity to connect with the progress they've made.

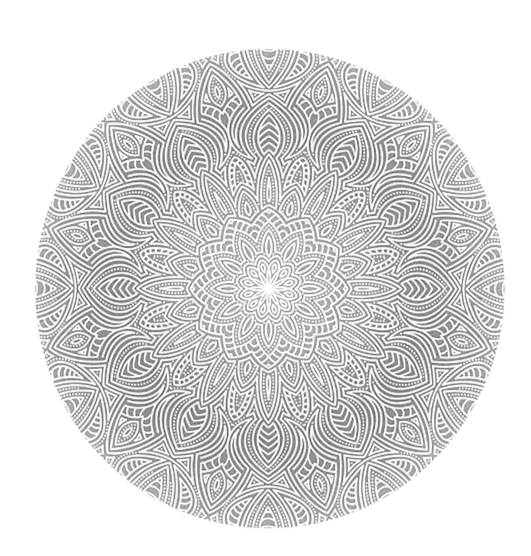

Samādhi

The final session of MYACT turns toward the topics of death, grief, and saying good-bye. In India, preparing for death is the very purpose of yoga. Patañjali's Yoga Sūtras posit that yoga's final destination is *samādhi*, a meditative consciousness in which the seer returns to where they once came from. Arguably, this is a place of self-acceptance that the seer has never left but may have forgotten. Said more simply, samādhi is to become fully absorbed, to die. Although this topic may sound morbid, it is full immersion that allows the seer to begin their journey again, taking proverbial stock of their life and journeying through each process, endlessly, until their time is over. This final session prepares participants to make sense of their future painful experiences, and even their dying time, through self-acceptance.

Ending a relationship can in itself be a difficult topic for participants. Allow an extra amount of time to discuss, debrief, and process what saying good-bye means to each participant. Again, we hesitate to call functional self-disclosure a necessity, but in our experience, it's essential to the facilitator position. Consider sharing your own feelings and reactions about the group ending.

Beginning Meditation: Death

We begin this meditation with a short period of silence and ring a bell or singing bowl, or both, for one to two minutes before leading the group through the meditation.

> This is our final session.
>
> Take a breath and notice whatever experience shows up for you. Be curious. What thoughts, feelings, and memories show up around saying good-bye?
>
> Whatever you notice showing up, we wish to pose this thought for you to meditate on: Grief is the love you feel for that which you've lost. And love is the grief you have for that which you have not yet lost.

Tim Gordon, founder of this practice, spent time in India, where a yoga teacher challenged him to think differently about what yoga means. The guru asked him, with all the research he had been doing, the books and articles he'd read, the ayurvedic clinics he'd visited, the endless discussions he'd had, what he thought the purpose of yoga was. Despite several answers that he personally thought cut to the heart of what yoga means, the guru insisted that Tim had missed the point. Tim paused and humbly deferred to the guru, who, in response, said only "death."

In India, some yoga teachers instruct students to find Savasana, the final resting posture, by saying, "Prepare to die." And rather than completing the practice with the soft ring of a bell or the invitation to wake the body gently, the teacher drops a heavy block or snaps a piece of wood, signaling the moment for the yogis to resume daily life.

Throughout this group, session after session, we've invited you to find Savasana at the beginning of our sessions as a way to give in to the moment, letting go of what comes through the door with you in order to make our practice space sacred, a place where we slow down with one another and prepare our heart, body, and mind to let go. Sometimes we focused on letting go of our attachment to outcomes. In this final group, our theme is complete absorption into our experience, saying good-bye to this group and sacred space. In short, we could say, "Prepare to die."

We end this beginning Savasana by dropping a wood block on the ground and then wait for participants to sit up and join us at the front of their mats.

Before transitioning into the debrief, take a long pause and make eye contact with each participant, if doing so feels appropriate, and say, "Today is about saying good-bye. We're going to connect with the skills we've learned and the relationships we've grown, both with ourselves and each other. Sometimes life requires us to say good-bye or to move forward. We should approach this process as we do all other experiences in life: with attention and intention.

Group Dialogue: Debriefing Home Practice

Debriefing the home practice is an opportunity to talk about how it went for participants, to reinforce their engagement in new behaviors, and also to troubleshoot problems that may have arisen. We like to use these questions as prompts:

Before we move on, how did everyone feel after they went home last week?

Did you have any difficulty or success monitoring and modifying your sleep habits?

How was it to do this practice?

What did you notice while doing it?

Looking at the Sleep Tracker worksheet data, did you notice any patterns?

Did you commit yourself to any values-based action this week?

How did it go?

Reflection on Session One's Intention-Setting Exercise

We now return to the intention-setting exercise from session one. Either re-create the whiteboard the group generated in that first session, if you took a picture of it, or return to participants the pieces of paper on which they wrote their hoped outcomes, or intentions, from the group. Invite each group member to share their reflection upon seeing their intentions again. It's not abnormal for many participants' expectations to have changed from the first group session. MYACT poses a noneliminative agenda that violates the convention of reducing pain, or eliminating difficult thoughts and emotions, that most participants may have had at the beginning of the protocol. Specifically ask them if they received what they felt they needed at the beginning of the group. They may not have, but they may have gotten what they really needed from the group: a new way forward.

Yoga Is Dying

Historically in India, yoga as well as meditation are used to prepare for death. This is why the final posture of Savasana translates as Corpse Pose. With this pose and this practice, we're not preparing for death in the literal sense, rather we're practicing how to be present within the process of letting go. In this group, we have shared ourselves with others, held the pain of our group members, supported each other, and created strong connections, both participant to participant and facilitator to participant. While this group has given a lot to each person, the act of ending the group can feel like a loss to some. This session centers on the process of letting go and, in the case of this group, saying good-bye.

You'll now conduct the final yoga sequence, comprising the following practices:

- Standing Full-Sun Salutations

- Linking Warrior 1, Warrior 2, Triangle, Side Angle

- Bridge

- Freestyle Movement

- Supported Lying Twists

- Legs Up the Wall

Begin by completing a series of **Standing Full-Sun Salutations**, as described in session seven, and then link the standing poses of **Warrior 1**, **Warrior 2**, **Triangle**, and **Side Angle**, as described in session five. You might guide participants through this sequence once or twice, and then have them do one to three self-guided rounds. We often hold each pose for a couple of breaths in the first round before linking them together breath by breath, which is commonly how participants practice flows. After everyone has finished with this flow, lead the group through **Bridge**, as described in session three.

Freestyle Movement

Before moving into the cool-down postures, offer participants the opportunity to use the proprioception they've been cultivating throughout the protocol. This time of free movement is just a chance for them to tune in to how they're feeling, physically, mentally and emotionally, and to move in any way that feels good and expresses those feelings nonverbally. This part of the yoga session can even take the form of students doing some of their favorite postures or movements from the protocol. The freestyle movement can last from one to three minutes, depending on time or response from participants.

After the Freestyle Movement, it's time to cool down. Complete a series of **Supported Lying Twists**, as described in session one, and **Legs Up the Wall**, as described in session three.

Group Dialogue: Debriefing Yoga Practice

Encourage participants to sit at the front of their yoga mats in a seated posture that's comfortable for them: "Moving in your own time, find yourself seated at the front of your mat." You can then debrief the practice by asking the following prompts:

What did you notice in that practice?

What was it like to choose your own postures?

What did you notice in your experience that led to the postures you practiced?

Did you get hooked or find yourself looking to others to see what they were doing?

Zen Death Poem Readings

Ask each participant to read their Zen death poem aloud. If there are two facilitators, we've found it helpful for one of the facilitators to go first, and for the other facilitator to read theirs aloud last. End the exercise by asking each participant to share a few words about what they're feeling in the moment.

Saying Good-Bye Group Exercise

This group exercise is lengthy, but in our experience, it's impactful and meaningful for participants. In advance of the last session, we recommend that you make a schedule. It should list pairings of the participants, including the facilitators, such that everyone has an opportunity to say good-bye to each person. You might transition into the exercise with this: "Saying good-bye—endings in general—can be hard for a lot people, bringing up feelings of loss, sadness, and grief. This final group exercise is an invitation to come in contact with the pain that might show up for you as you take the time to connect with each person and say good-bye."

Tell them that they'll be meeting in pairs, and that by the end of the session, they'll have had a chance to meet with every person, including the facilitators, and that each person will have three minutes to speak before a bell will sound, indicating the speaker and listener should switch roles. We prefer to then announce who they'll be partnered with first based on the schedule, but you may wish to have them self-select.

Ring a bell to begin, and say, "Take three minutes to share something you appreciated or found meaningful about your partner's presence in this group, perhaps something they said or did. Finish by sharing your hopes for your partner in the future. After three minutes, I'll ring the bell so you can switch roles."

Set a timer for three minutes, and ring a bell when the three minutes have passed, saying, "It's now time to swap roles. Take three minutes to share something you appreciated or found meaningful about your partner's presence in this group, perhaps something they said or did. Finish by sharing what your hopes are for your partner in the future. After three minutes, I'll ring the bell and we'll change partners."

Session Eight Home Practice: Intentional Commitment to Whole Health

Take time in the final session to reflect on the progress participants have made, but also turn toward the future to provide encouragement for staying the course and to normalize the process of living, which inevitably includes barriers, setbacks, and missteps. For this last exercise, have them write a letter to their future self in which they highlight their values and specific actions they're taking now—and hope to be taking in the future—to set them on a meaningful path forward. Ask them to also identify any potential barriers or setbacks, external or internal, and discuss how they'll meet these challenges while staying committed to what matters. Additionally, encourage them to describe their experience of the MYACT protocol and what key points have stuck with them.

This letter serves as a commitment to themselves as well as the whole health model. It also provides them a brief, easy-to-digest, personalized letter they can turn to whenever they find themselves caught up in old unworkable patterns or problematic habits. This is the home practice: to refer to the letter when the going gets tough. If time permits, we ask each person to share their letter aloud. If time is limited, we may ask if anyone is interested in reading theirs out loud to the group.

Ending Savasana or Seated Meditation: Saying Good-Bye

In this final meditation for the group, you can use the following script or, as with all interventions in this book, modify it for the context of your group and the topics you've covered. In our MYACT groups, we add one "good-bye" comment during the meditation for each participant based on their progress in the group. This comment is individualized for the participant and focused on either reinforcing a new behavior they've engaged in or validating something they've struggled with.

In India, this posture of Savasana is practiced just as we are doing it now, at the end of yoga practice. I've used the Sanskrit name in this room because its direct translation—Corpse or Dead Body Pose—is not so welcoming.

In India, some yoga teachers instruct their class to take this final relaxation pose by saying, "Prepare to die."

Although this might seem jarring, this final pose is the ultimate act of detachment, putting us in the mind-set of letting go; of making peace with our unrequited love, our unfulfilled dreams, our unmet goals; of surrendering to the divine, eternal infinity that we once came from and now awaits each of us.

In our last moments of this final session, with a deep sense of gratitude for your commitment to this work and dedication to practice, and with respect for what we've cocreated in this space, I ask you to prepare yourself now for your dying time. Lay in this final pose. Don't turn your attention away, but instead bring your focus fully into whatever occurs to you here and now.

After participants have been in Savasana an amount of time that seems appropriate, invite them to introduce movement to their body and come to a seated position at the top of their mat. Then end the final session of MYACT as you ended session one and all the others, with chanting, sharing appreciations, and a closing posture.

Working with Individuals

- All of the exercises in session eight can be modified to be a one-on-one interaction. The goal of this last session is to process saying good-bye, highlight progress made, and prepare the client for the future. This can be done as one large, fluid conversation or it can be broken up into distinct parts, as is done in the group protocol. The choice, as always, is yours.

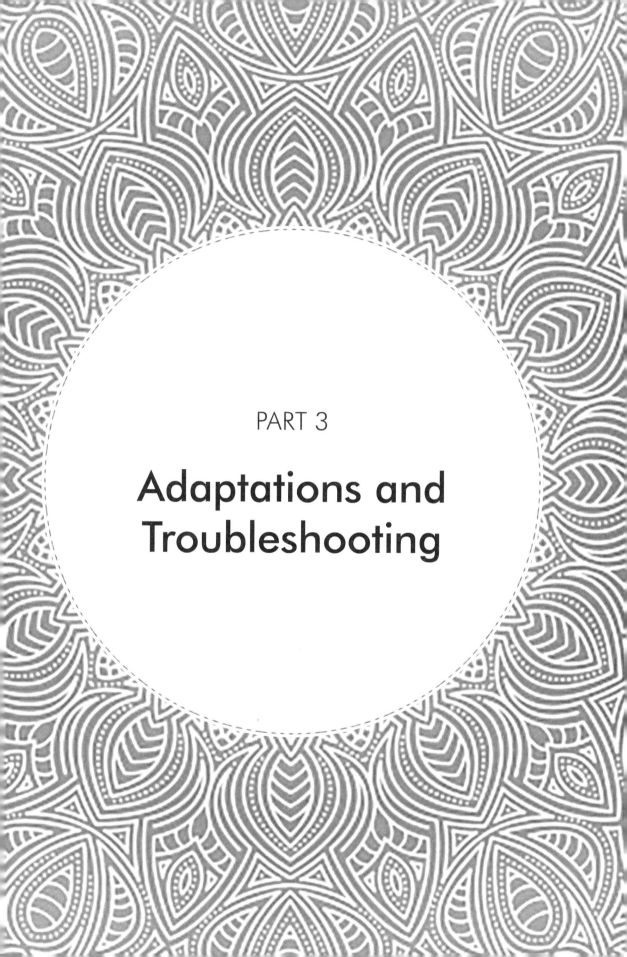

PART 3

Adaptations and Troubleshooting

While it may seem like we covered all there possibly could be to cover regarding MYACT, there is still more we'd like to impart. We understand that not everyone will run the MYACT protocol as described in part two, rather they'll use the concepts and scripts and poses to enhance the good work they're already doing. Within this context, we feel it important to explore some additional relevant information in this final part of the book.

Chapter four explores how both mental health professionals and yoga teachers can incorporate MYACT into their settings and use it with individual clients. Chapter five covers scope of practice considerations for non-mental-health professionals. We are aware that yoga teachers often are the first line of contact for people seeking mental health treatment. It's one of the reasons we decided to write this book. This reality can lead to tricky situations in which yoga teachers find themselves wanting to help but not wanting to step outside their area of expertise. We explore how to navigate these challenges, as well as discuss practices that may be common in the yoga community but are harmful and not supported by science. We conclude with a discussion of what your next steps might be, armed with information about MYACT in mind, as you close this book and more forward.

CHAPTER 4

Weaving MYACT into Individual Therapy Sessions

This chapter is all about finding that sweet spot in which you can integrate MYACT into your practice setting. We encourage everyone to read both sections, even though only one likely applies to you, because understanding how others work can provide insight.

Mental Health Professionals

Though our eight-week group protocol is comprehensive and effective, we understand that a large portion of therapeutic work is individual work. The same is true for our own practices. When working individually, we roughly follow the eight-session progression of yoga practices you've read about, but we have a much more fluid process-based way of addressing participant issues. This means that we tailor each individual session to the presenting problem of the participant, rather than using predetermined exercises and topics. Tim and Jessica cover practicing ACT with a process-based focus in *The ACT Approach* (Gordon & Borushok 2017).

We use yoga poses in the majority of the work we do. Even clients who respond to more traditional, seated forms of mindfulness practice can benefit from contact with an active form of mindfulness. It helps to show them that this practice is not relegated to quiet, still moments only. We choose to introduce yoga when a client has a hard time being grounded in session, is regularly distracted by thoughts, or struggles to be in contact with the present moment in session (for example, someone who is rambling or tangential).

Before we introduce yoga to these clients, we validate that the thoughts, feelings, sensations, and memories they're struggling with are very real and very difficult. We may use the life map or traditional talk therapy to address the problems with trying to escape, avoid, or control these private experiences, ending in a place where clients recognize there is no delete key for their pain. Once we have that platform established, we might introduce the idea of trying yoga like this:

> So what I'd like to work with you on is changing how you interact with the painful stuff that shows up in your life, since we now know that trying to get rid of it doesn't work. There's research showing that the majority of people are thinking about something other than what they're doing the majority of the time.
>
> Imagine you're on autopilot and not thinking about what you're doing. If you begin experiencing something unpleasant, you're not thinking about what it's like to carry it or what the costs of fighting it are. Now imagine this tissue box is something painful. [*Show the client a tissue box.* We may then gently throw the tissue box toward them for them to catch, asking, "Did you choose to catch it?" Clients often respond, "No, I just reacted."]
>
> Now, I want you to notice what happens when you encounter something painful and choose to hold it, when you're aware of the pain showing up. [*Hand the client the tissue box.*] Did you notice a difference? I want to show you some practices so you are better able to notice what shows up and then have the freedom to choose what you do next rather than simply reacting. [The client can set the tissue box down now].
>
> We're going to try a lot of different things to see what works for you. Remember, our work is not about the specific practice; it's about learning a certain way of noticing what works for you so you are better able to interrupt the patterns of avoidance that aren't working for you and instead choose a behavior that does. Some people discover they really enjoy meditation, whereas others really enjoy yoga, tai chi, or other strategies. Let's see what works for you. I'd like to introduce you to some different types of mindfulness, both traditional eyes-closed meditation and some seated yoga poses. Would you be willing to give them a try?

Often we introduce mindfulness, or noticing, as a seated, eyes-closed mindfulness exercise, and nine times out of ten, the exercise lands well with the client. Some people may struggle with focusing their attention; others may have had a bad experience with meditation, hold a stereotype about it, or may not be interested in it. In these cases, we use yoga to get at the same noticing processes. As we said previously, even clients who do well with seated mindfulness may benefit from yoga, as it shatters the myth that mindfulness can only be achieved in stillness.

Sometimes yoga poses are a structured part of a session, and we begin or end the session with a yoga pose similar to how we might use a mindfulness exercise to settle into a session or end a session. Sometimes yoga arises more fluidly, say if we notice a client getting caught up in emotions or distracted. For example, if a client is crying hysterically, losing their train of thought regularly, reporting feeling overwhelmed, or rambling, we may check in and ask permission to interrupt them. Most clients respond positively to this approach. We can then comment on what we noticed happening in the room or even on our own experience: "I noticed we're both talking very quickly," or "I noticed we've gotten a little off topic. Is it okay if we pause for a moment here and just reconnect with what we're experiencing in a different way?"

A good pose to start with is Seated Sun Salutation, because it's not physically taxing for most and is done seated, which may feel safer or less unusual for a client in a therapy setting. There is, however, no rule or protocol for which yoga poses should be used in individual sessions. You can start with easier yoga poses and build to more complex ones, as we outlined in the MYACT protocol, or try something else. The most important consideration is meeting your client with the right yoga pose.

Clients who are anxious often have difficulty slowing down. Yoga may make them feel vulnerable or threatened, so starting with a slower pose can help set the tone of the session. Beginning with Seated Sun Salutation to meet their pace might be a good option, and then using Savasana and restorative postures, such as Supported Lying Twist, to help them slow down and cool down.

Clients who are depressed or have flat affect can struggle with engagement. It might help to begin with Seated Sun Salutation to match their pace, and then transition into postures that challenge strength, such as Warrior 1 and Warrior 2. This progression helps engage clients and put them in tune with their body because they have to focus when doing these strength poses. It is important to give them specific cues of where to look or what to notice.

Clients who are dysregulated, are emotionally volatile, struggle with trauma memories, or often express anger may benefit from slow poses. For example, you could begin with one of the Sun Salutations, or Side Angle, and exaggerate the movements. Cues such as "Take the entire length of an inhale to raise your arms," or "Notice the emotional quality of being in this moment," can draw attention to the experience and help the client slow down rather that react or be caught up in the chaos of thoughts or emotions. Always end with a long period of restorative practice to slow them down and to get them more focused on actual sensations rather than feared, imagined sensations. For example, while lying in Savasana, you could say to the client, "Trace an outline of your body with your mind."

You can also use yoga as a discrimination task, to train the client to notice what it's like to do one action or another. This is similar to what we ask of people when we do the life map. For example, starting in Child's Pose, you could ask clients to notice the quality of their breath and how much strain there is in the body as their knees press into the floor. After four or five breaths, have them transition into Table and either press back into plank or into a harder variation of Table in which they lift their left arm and right leg. Then ask, "If I asked you to stay in this posture for seven more breaths, how would you react? Would you drop down into Child's Pose, lower your arm and leg, or keep your arm and leg extended? And if you stay in this more difficult pose, what's it about for you? What are you reacting to?" This helps clients tune in to their motivations for behavior. Is it driven by avoidance of painful experiences or thoughts or rigid rules, or is it guided by what's important to them in that moment? The goal here is for them simply to notice what's driving them.

We often give clients yoga poses as home practices, just as we'd give them exercises for practicing mindfulness. The goal is the same with both: noticing.

Before we close, we'd like to briefly mention consent and trauma sensitivity. Make sure you always let clients know what the yoga poses will look like before beginning, so they can accurately choose whether to participate or not. Avoid physical contact with clients when doing yoga, especially in initial sessions. You'll still have the ability to make adjustments or provide demonstrations, but these don't need to include touching. Even if you're practicing in the context that both client and therapist are equals, know that you're in a position of power. You need to be extremely careful to not accidentally put someone in a position that makes them uncomfortable, because in the end, they believe you're the expert.

After the first couple of sessions, you may choose to have a direct conversation about touching. This may include a discussion about trying more challenging yoga poses and comfort level with adjustments. Make sure you always let your client know that saying no is a completely acceptable response, and that you can stick to giving verbal directions only. Some clients may feel they need to say yes to get the full experience. This is not true. Even if clients do give permission for physical adjustments, always ask before providing any. This means getting an explicit response (yes) and making it very clear that saying no is okay. You can use hand gestures to guide people without touching them or demonstrate the pose yourself. A client may be generally okay with touch but feel particularly vulnerable in certain poses or during certain sessions.

And finally, never stand behind clients, as that may seem threatening to people who have experienced trauma or feel particularly vulnerable. We don't mean to be alarmists. We just want clients and therapists alike to have safe and helpful sessions. If you use proper ethical and clinical judgment, you'll provide your clients with a new tool for living a meaningful life.

Yoga Instructors

As a yoga teacher, you may already be working with clients individually, or you may be looking to extend your practice to include private clients. Regardless of where you are in your career, the following information provides an informed framework for the work you're going to be doing with clients.

So why might someone contact a yoga instructor for an individual session? Clients may book private sessions for a number of reasons: they have physical concerns (chronic pain, athletes with tightness or form issues), want to take yoga practice to the next level, desire targeted one-on-one practices (mindfulness). During an initial intake, consider asking questions about why they're here, and create a body map to identify any physical issues regardless of whether they're what the client identified as a focus. Clients may come with a variety of concerns, and it's important to isolate what is the most important to begin focusing on.

The intake is a great opportunity to bring values into the work you do. For example, if a person comes in complaining of pain or tightness in the hip, you might ask, "What would it mean for you to have better function in your hips? What would that allow you to do?" The answers not only offer insight into the client's personal values, but they help increase the client's motivation to continue with the work even when it becomes difficult. You might even go further and identify potential barriers to your work together up front in an effort to address issues before beginning your work together: "What are some of the things you feel or think might get in the way of you committing to this practice or practicing in a kinder way?"

The next step is to provide a clear picture about the type of work you'll be doing and to get buy-in from the client, and for them to provide informed consent. We often explain that our method doesn't focus on excessively long deep breathing, but rather on letting the breath breathe itself. More importantly, we explain how we're going to be using the breath as a feedback tool for checking in with the body and mind during movement. You might use the example of feeling anxious and holding your breath: "We might not always realize how we're feeling, but our breath can give us insight into how our body and mind are working or feeling." Oftentimes, clients come in to use yoga to address physical concerns and don't realize the connection between their body and mental health concerns.

It might be more challenging to get buy-in from clients who have a background in yoga. It's harder for them to defuse, or get space, from the ideas they have about what certain poses or practices should be like. Their past training makes it more difficult to approach the work we do with a beginner's mind. When we come across this challenge, we intentionally pay more attention to exploring different perspectives and creating openness with the goal of fostering willingness to give this work, this way, a try. Be careful of getting drawn into a debate or of creating too firm of a wall. People often become defensive when they feel their beliefs are being challenged, regardless of how rational the argument. It's important that we, too, are flexible in how we interact with clients and highlight how the work we're doing can build upon the foundation the client already has: "Sometimes we need to break something down in order to build it back up again."

Similarly, athletes who are used to more vigorous practices may reject the protocol, thinking that the poses, movements, and noticing activities are too easy and won't help. With clients like this, validate their concerns that this work may not be a vigorous or physically demanding practice, but highlight what they can gain from it. You might say something like this:

What if we stay open to the idea that this could work? Is it okay for you to try this to see if it works? Is there something in the program you found difficult attention-wise rather than physically challenging? Maybe for you, this work isn't purely about a physically demanding practice, rather the way it helps you is by improving your connection to your body and how it's functioning. This connection might help you move more in sync with your body, listening and adjusting based on its feedback.

For individuals who are experiencing pain, your work should focus on choosing poses and movements based on biomechanical needs. That training exceeds the scope of this book; however, there has been extensive research on the benefits of yoga therapy in terms of treating physical concerns or injuries. What MYACT brings to working with these clients is awareness. We emphasize that individuals with chronic pain should focus on feeling the breath. Consider beginning each session with a breathing exercise with the goal of increasing awareness of how the breath moves through the body and how the individual experiences the body as a whole. Individuals with chronic pain can develop habits, such as holding their breath or holding their body in rigid postures, as ways to brace against the pain. These strategies are ineffective and often lead to a rigidity that can increase the chance of further injury because the body doesn't move flexibly.

In fact, when we begin a session with a first-time client (or in MYACT groups), we'll say something to the effect of this: "In this particular style of practice, we want you to try and move in a way that doesn't create discomfort or pain or increase the discomfort or pain that you might already be walking into the room with." Then, begin with the breath so they can develop that skill separate from movement, folding their attention and breathing practices into movement and poses as their skills build.

In all clients, you should look for cues of rigidity: Are they holding their breath in this position? Did a visibly noticeable amount of tension start to arise somewhere in the body? You don't want to simply point it out; instead, help people recognize it on their own and begin to notice what is happening in that moment. Many people aren't even aware that their breath or body is displaying signs of stress, anxiety, discomfort, or pain. If a client's body begins to tense up in unnecessary ways, we recommend against just asking the client to relax or soften. Ask if they can feel that their body or breath has shifted, then take steps to try and change the behavior. You might even get them to do a movement a few times in a row so they have a chance to feel the change in their body or breath happening. Remember, the goal is to provide tools and practices that they can take with them and use in their life.

How we approach teaching, though, not what we teach, is one of the best ways we can help our clients. Even though we have an underlying philosophy to guide our practice, everyone's body is different. We often try to come up with a thing or process that works for everyone, and the truth is it just doesn't. We must always come back to function: How does this pose work for this person? We don't take a structured, prescriptive approach in MYACT because it's not relevant for asanas, nor is it the way you cue movement. It's good practice to have decent cues to use regularly to instruct movement or positioning; however, we encourage you to challenge yourself to develop different ways of cuing or explaining things to clients so you are prepared for their individuality.

For example, consider teaching a client to do a particular crunching-type movement. The aim is to get the client to tighten the abdomen so the distance between the ribs and hips becomes shorter. Let's say you use a cue that works for the majority of clients: "Can you feel your abdominals contracting? Can you feel that when your abdominals contract, your ribs are closer to your hips?" What if the client says they can't? Perhaps you can tell the instruction is confusing to the client, so you take a different approach: "Put your hands on your belly. Do you notice that if you tighten your abdomen, your fingers get closer?" Again, the client struggles with this cue.

Instead of rushing on to a different cue or becoming frustrated with the client for not understanding, take a step back to think through how you might help this client understand what you're highlighting. "Is it okay to go back to your breath for a moment? I want to think about where to go next." This is a simple statement, but it's one that can be hard for a lot of yoga teachers because they fear they'll look incompetent or unsure of what to do next. But the goal is to help the client, not to appear brilliant, and sometimes that means acknowledging you're stuck or confused or need to think something through.

By taking this approach, we're also modeling psychological flexibility to clients. We are showing them that it's okay to slow down sometimes and take a step back before moving forward again. During the breathing break, you might have the space to recognize that all the cues you'd given were related to the abdomen and thus try a different perspective: "When you tighten your abs, do you notice your shoulder blades lifting off the floor? And when you feel that contraction, do you feel your low spine get closer to the floor?" If you're willing to acknowledge that your cuing may be the issue, and if you're open to pausing and looking at the issue from a different perspective, more often than not, you'll be successful in communicating with your clients.

It is your responsibility to find the appropriate language to communicate with your client. If a client isn't getting something we're talking about, it's not the client's fault, it's the way we are approaching the topic. We need to take a different perspective or use a different metaphor or example to help the client understand. This will not only cut down on a lot of your frustration, but it will expand the way you view the body as it forces you to become more creative and see movement from multiple perspectives. The more you practice perspective taking, the more variation in cues you'll develop and the better you'll be able to help your clients.

It's important to always give home practices. It could be a breathing exercise or a series of movements. To develop relevant home practice, we recommend asking clients what progress and success mean to them. Remind them that you're not a teacher who's going to grade them or fail them if they don't do their homework: "It's not that I want you to feel guilty if you don't do your home practice. Home practice is about taking steps toward getting what you want out of this work. The more you do the home practice, the more you're moving toward what you want." In terms of frequency, you might say this: "There are seven days in a week, so aim for five. If you hit three, that's okay." Stating goals like this immediately cuts down on behaviors such as lying about how many days they did the practice or if they did the practice at all. Also, some clients may know that they can't do seven days of practice and thus simply give up. Telling them ahead of time that seven days of practice isn't required may encourage them to engage in the behaviors we're looking for.

At the end of the day, instructing yoga with individual clients is all about being flexible to what shows up in the room. Don't make assumptions about how the practice will function, and be sure to practice a willingness to let go of rigid schedules. Be comfortable with not knowing what will happen next. Sometimes we may want a certain outcome from a practice, but never forget to listen to the client. If we're too stuck on a particular outcome, we can miss how the practice is actually functioning for the client. Rather than assuming how something feels for a client, always inquire: "Does that feel better, worse, or neutral?" Or, "How does that feel for you?"

And above all, remind yourself why you love this work. It can be hard to learn new things and even harder to implement them. Be kind to yourself, and stay committed to your work and aware of what about it drives you. Day by day, this new approach will lead to a change in how you view the world and how you help your clients.

CHAPTER 5

Scope of Practice Considerations for Non-Mental-Health Professionals

Like practitioners in other healing professions, yoga teachers often find themselves in awkward positions, wanting to help those who come to them without crossing any ethical lines. This chapter is devoted to exploring what those lines are and how yoga teachers can navigate difficult situations, both within yoga class and outside of it. We'll explore strategies and approaches to navigating scope of practice, and we'll conclude by highlighting some of the worst practices that have found their way into mainstream yoga culture and can cause significant harm.

What to Do

The main tools yoga instructors work with are breath, movement, and stillness. The focus of your work centers around understanding whether clients need more or less of these three things, and then guiding them through the process of tuning in to themselves.

When people come into contact with the present moment and experience unpleasant thoughts, feelings, sensations, and memories, they may react in class. A common scenario involves cuing the class or an individual client to bring attention to the body or a certain movement, and there's a strong reaction (for example, a person leaves the room or has an emotional outburst, such as crying). Because this happens in a yoga context, it's natural for the client to reach out for advice on what to do. As the instructor, it's important to normalize the experience, making clear that increasing awareness can sometimes bring us into contact with unpleasant experiences. Emphasize that whatever happened was not disruptive to you or the class, and that they are free to do whatever they need to in that moment. For example, a client who leaves the room or goes back into Child's Pose while the rest of the class carries on with the practice may feel embarrassed by their action or worry that it was distracting. If a participant asks for advice, a helpful response might be something like this:

> There are so many variables at play that it's hard to say what the underlying issue could be, and it's outside of my field of expertise to try and figure it out. My job is not to pinpoint what's going on, but rather to give you more tools for exploring the issue. You might consider doing some research on what happened [perhaps suggest a book or an article]. And if you'd like to talk to someone who is more specialized than me, I'd be happy to refer you to someone in the community who I know is qualified to answer your questions or help you find answers.

Sometimes the person won't seek you out for advice. In these instances, it may be helpful to casually—and not in front of others—say, "I just wanted to check in. I noticed that you had a reaction in class. Are you doing okay?" Keep in mind that the participant may not want to talk about what happened, and we don't want to force them to talk about something that was clearly troubling or upsetting to them. The participant's body language or how quickly they pack up after class may communicate to you that they don't want to be approached. Use your judgment to determine whether it would be helpful to check in or not.

If a reaction happens in an individual session, you may want to casually check in: "Is this something that you want to talk about? Is this something you need assistance with? If so, we can talk about it." This is where the life map or general ACT language about pain can be helpful for exploring what happened in that moment for the client. While it's helpful to be aware of potential referral options in your community, do not recommend that a client talk to someone or seek professional help if they don't bring it up. Whether you want it or not, you have influence over your clients. You must be careful not to pressure them into something they're not ready for under the guise of helping.

If you do end up providing referrals for individual clients, consider getting a release of information so you can coordinate care with the specialist. The client must be the source of this release, which gives you and the specialist permission to discuss the client with each other. This access to information is often helpful. Specialists may provide recommendations for poses, body parts, or breathing techniques, including what to build up to, avoid, or emphasize based on your area of expertise and the client's needs. With that information, you're then able to create a protocol that not only meets the client's needs for yoga practice but does so in a way that assists their mental health needs.

Another opportunity for collaboration is to run the eight-week MYACT protocol with mental health professionals. This joint effort allows each of you to focus on your strengths and scope of practice during the protocol while also expanding your knowledge. You get to see first-hand how the therapist answers and addresses certain issues, allowing you to become more familiar with the other tools that are available for helping clients, and vice versa.

And finally, we cannot rely on blog posts or other news outlets with flashy headlines to provide us with an accurate state of the evidence regarding yoga and mental health. Although you don't need to know every last bit of research on physical and mental health practices, it's helpful to stay up-to-date on functional information that you can use to improve your practice and teachings. Resources such as Google Scholar are excellent places to gain access to peer-reviewed journal articles. Blog and news outlets often misrepresent, overstate, or misinterpret data in order simplify or sensationalize results; for these reasons, it's best to stick to peer-reviewed journal articles. They may be less fun to read, but they provide a more accurate picture of what is known from a scientific perspective. And be sure to read the actual articles and not just the abstracts. As a yoga teacher, you may be astounded by some of the practices researchers count as "yoga." The methods section of an article will give you a step-by-step outline of what the researchers actually did to create their study, and it may clarify what they considered "yoga."

Don't fret! You've got this. Now that we've covered helpful practices and approaches to client mental health concerns, let's take a look at some of the ways we can overstep our bounds or use misguided information in harmful ways.

What Not to Do

Pain is often a primary focus in yoga practice. However, while there is mounting evidence for the benefits of yoga in managing chronic pain, some beliefs about pain can send incorrect and harmful messages to clients. Consider an instructor who approaches yoga as a way to correlate pain in certain areas of the body with different samskāras (scars in your life). This approach is not based on any empirical evidence and can be harmful, because the instructor is placing blame in ways that have no option for resolution and create problems where there are none.

For example, what if a person attends yoga classes due to tight hips from running often, and the teacher suggests that tight hips reflect conflict with a female in this person's life. Based on these unfounded assumptions, this person may interact differently with female loved ones or see conflict where there is none. Meanwhile, they're not doing the practices that can relieve tension in their hips. Therefore, not only is the instructor introducing conflict in the person's life, they're also failing to address the participant's actual issue—the thing that a yoga teacher's skills can actually help with.

On a similar note, be careful of protocols that claim to be "yoga therapy." While yoga therapy as a practice for addressing physical conditions has scientific backing, some protocols that purport to provide therapeutic healing don't always have the background and credentials to appropriately teach these skills. Yoga therapy is a relatively young concept, and not all of its teachings are backed by research. Unfortunately, many yoga teachers read the research about how yoga is good for anxiety or depression but don't stop to understand the mechanics that lead to positive outcomes. What this means is they're often operating with limited or incorrect knowledge. This is not only potentially harmful, but it also raises legal concerns. Though there is no board or regulatory body that oversees scope of practice for yoga instructors, you can still put yourself at risk of litigation should your work cause harm. That is why we created clear guidelines to follow in MYACT, which we presented in this book, and encourage you to learn about mental health only from actual mental health professionals.

Along these lines, clients may share non-yoga-related personal information and difficulties with you and ask for your help. Though it can be helpful to give home practice to bring more attention to certain struggles or concerns, such as the Mapping Your Life or Know Your Hooks worksheets, please be wary of offering advice or trying to fix their problem. As an instructor, you're in a position of power and authority, and people can take your offhanded comments or suggestions as informed advice they should follow. Take the time to get to know your community so you have people you trust to recommend to clients.

Another reason why offering advice or trying to problem solve can be risky is that what works for you may not work for everyone. If we begin to offer personal anecdotes as the truth and the only way forward, we may be cutting clients off from information that could help them and creating a sense of failure or self-defeat if they don't have success or find relief after following our instruction. A good rule of thumb is to only share personal anecdotes with clients when asked. It can also be helpful to talk about practices you've tried that didn't work in order to emphasize that life is a journey, and it's the responsibility of clients to try different strategies for themselves to see what works for them. A good way to phrase your experience is to say, "This works for me, but it may not work for you. Let's try it and see how it works for you."

The goal is to not emphasize only one particular approach to healing. There are many ways that a person can walk their own journey. As beneficial as yoga is, it has potential negative side effects. For example, clients can use yoga as a way to escape something they don't want to feel or deal with rather than use it as an opportunity to become more aware of the present moment and all of their experiences. We outline these ethical dilemmas and considerations not to scare you away from trying something new or helping someone in need, but rather to encourage you to explore the situations you find yourself in and how you handle them. This process will make you better at identifying when you can help and when you should refer clients to another resource.

Continuing Your Journey with MYACT

It is our hope that by now, you're as excited as we are about the boundless possibilities inherent in this work. We've walked with you on this journey through the wisdom and traditions of yoga and ACT, gotten technical with relational frame theory and basic anatomy, and laid out session by session how to bring this protocol to life. As we come to an end, we want to reiterate that strict adherence to the MYACT protocol is not a requirement for bringing this work into yours. Rather, MYACT purports a truth, a blending of ideas. It approaches healing and emotional balance supported by science, but it remains flexible to the details of life and to life's context. And in its very nature, MYACT is active.

MYACT is a blending of ACT and yoga, but it's so much more than the sum of its parts. While ACT adds context to the prescriptive wisdom traditions of yoga to create more flexibility and autonomy in how clients approach life, yoga adds techniques and practices that can reach those who don't respond to seated meditation or talk therapy or who are interested in a novel, less stigmatized way of healing. Yoga is an experiential way of teaching ACT through movement, yet MYACT bridges the two worlds of science and tradition, creating an opportunity to reach those who belong to one or the other, don't fit in either, or belong to both, bringing some peace and balance to their world. If you understand the components that make up MYACT and the approach as a whole, you'll be able to make MYACT your own, bring it to life in your practice, and reach nearly anyone. This is our greatest wish.

Yoga teachers, we hope you come away from this book knowing how to appropriately use yoga with people with mental health issues and which yoga practices are evidence based. No matter what emotional or psychological issues show up in your classes or individual sessions, we believe you'll be able to meet them with psychological flexibility, thereby helping clients reach emotional balance through the work you love. Mental health professionals, we hope you walk away understanding yoga practices and feeling confident enough to incorporate them into your current work and the eight-week MYACT protocol. We hope we've made clear how you can use the body to help clients connect with painful cognitive content in new ways and expand their behavioral repertoires, and reach clients who haven't responded to treatment.

We're so excited that you went on this journey with us. After the metaphorical "the end," we suggest you take some time to think through everything you've read. Examine it, refute it, explore it, and, finally, practice it. Beginning with small steps forward, create a plan for introducing MYACT to your clients. With each step, challenge yourself to move out of your comfort zone and into a place where growth, both yours and your clients, can flourish. *Mindful Yoga-Based Acceptance and Commitment Therapy* is not a book to be read once and displayed on a shelf; it's meant to be reread, underlined, tabbed, and generally lived. If you find yourself uncertain in your practice, refer back to the book. It is our sincere hope that after reading these pages and closing the book it isn't "the end"; rather, it's a continuation of your journey to bring mindful yoga into your practice.

If you want to take your practice to the next level, we offer a MYACT online course with video demonstrations through Praxis (http://www.praxiscet.com) and run MYACT yoga teacher trainings annually (at least we do at the time of this book's publication; check out http://www.yourpsychology.ca/yoga for more information). The teacher training is an immersive experience and well worth the effort, offering participants the chance to live the MYACT protocol. Having completed this two-hundred-hour training, you can then register as a yoga instructor with Yoga Alliance, an international nonprofit association that trains, supports, and protects the integrity of the yoga community. Both of these educational opportunities are great options to further your training and connect with others working toward the same end, but they are in no way a requirement. *Mindful Yoga-Based Acceptance and Commitment Therapy* is meant to provide you all the tools you need to be self-sufficient in offering MYACT.

This book has been a labor of love for the three of us. We spent countless hours over dinner and way too many drinks at Starbucks thinking, creating, and challenging ourselves to make this protocol and book something of value to yoga teachers and mental health professionals and the people they serve. In these pages we gave you a foundation, and now it's your turn to build upon it. And we really hope you do. Don't fear; you won't be alone. You are one of many on this journey, coming from different backgrounds, settings, and practices, but all with open hearts, flexible minds, and a passion for helping others achieve emotional balance.

We can't wait to see what you can achieve. Good luck!

References

Āranya, H. (1984). *Yoga philosophy of Patañjali: Containing his yoga aphorisms with Vyāsa's commentary in Sanskrit and a translation with annotations including many suggestions for the practice of yoga.* Albany, NY: State University of New York Press.

AYI. Yoga-Sutra 1—Samadhi pada: About enlightenment. Accessed August 26, 2018. https://www.ashtangayoga.info/philosophy/yoga-sutra/chapter-1.

Clark, B. (2012). *The complete guide to Yin yoga: The philosophy and practice of Yin yoga.* Ashland, OR: White Cloud Press.

Eisendrath, S., Chartier, M., & McLane, M. (2011). Adapting mindfulness-based cognitive therapy for treatment-resistant depression: A clinical case study. *Cognitive and Behavioral Practice,* 18 (3), 362–370.

Feuerstein, G. (2008). *The yoga tradition: Its history, literature, philosophy, and practice.* Prescott, AZ: Hohm Press.

Gordon, T., & Borushok, J. (2017). *The ACT approach: A comprehensive guide for acceptance and commitment therapy.* Eau Claire, WI: PESI Publishing & Media.

Hayes, S. C., Luoma, J. B., Bond, F. W., Masuda, A., & Lillis, J. (2006). Acceptance and commitment therapy: Model, processes and outcomes. *Behaviour Research and Therapy, 44* (1), 1–25.

Miller, B. S. (1998). *Yoga: Discipline of freedom: The Yoga Sūtra attributed to Patañjali.* New York: Bantam.

Polk, K. L. (2014). The matrix, evolution, and improving work-group functioning with Ostrom's eight design principles. In K. L. Polk & B. Schoendorff (Eds.), *The ACT matrix: A new approach to building psychological flexibility across settings and populations.* Oakland, CA: New Harbinger.

Remski, M. (2012). *Threads of yoga: A remix of Patañjali's Sutras, with commentary and reverie.* Cork: BookBaby.

Stephens, M. (2010). *Teaching yoga: Essential foundations and techniques.* Berkeley, CA: North Atlantic.

Wilson, K. G. (2009). *Mindfulness for two: An acceptance and commitment therapy approach to mindfulness in psychotherapy.* Oakland, CA: New Harbinger.

Timothy Gordon, MSW, is a social worker in Canada, and an internationally recognized, peer-reviewed acceptance and commitment therapy (ACT) trainer. He specializes in treating attachment- and trauma-related disorders. Tim is also a yoga teacher who integrates movement and yoga practices into his work. Tim's research has included yoga as a mental health intervention, ACT for chronic pain, and ACT with neonatal intensive care units. Tim is passionate about empowering people in various settings to use ACT. He has worked with the Parliament of Canada, and is involved in bringing ACT to sub-Saharan African countries with his colleagues at Commit and Act. Gordon, along with Jessica Borushok, is award-winning coauthor of *The ACT Approach.*

Jessica Borushok, PhD, is a clinical psychologist specializing in health-related problems, including obesity, chronic pain, and coping with chronic medical conditions. In addition to clinical work, Jessica provides ACT trainings and program development internationally. She has conducted a National Institute of Occupational Safety and Health (NIOSH) grant-funded pilot randomized controlled trial exploring the impact of ACT on physical activity among sedentary workers, and consulted on a grant-funded program using ACT with parents of children in neonatal intensive care units.

Steve Ferrell, E-RYT, teaches yoga, Ayurveda, anatomy, biomechanics, meditation, and mindfulness practices nationally across Canada. Steve has been studying and practicing yoga and meditation for over a decade. Over this time, he has worked with many techniques from different lineages of yoga and Buddhism, as well as studying West-based psychological/behavioral perspectives. Steve is certified in integrative yoga therapy: a yoga school started by Joseph LePage, founder of the International Association of Yoga Therapists. He continues to study with notable figures in the field and is involved in ongoing research studies to see how yoga, meditation, and Ayurveda can help people primarily in the mental health field.

Index

connections, valuing, 134
consciousness in motion meditation, 128
consent of clients, 218
context: behaviors in, 10, 12; observer self and, 21
contextual behavioral science, 173
contextualscience.org website, 186
cool-down postures, 89
Corpse Pose. *See* Savasana practices
Cow Face pose, 63
creative hopelessness, 107
crown of the head, 28
cues: behavioral, 101; movement, 35–36; yoga, 176–177

D

Daily Commitment Questions Recording Form, 151
Dead Body Pose. *See* Savasana practices
death: beginning meditation on, 205–206; yoga as preparing for, 205, 206, 208
debriefing: ACT improve exercise, 166; beginning meditations, 81, 108, 133; bold move practice, 81–82; connecting to your future self, 186; Escape, Avoidance, and Control Checklist, 109; home practice, 81–82, 108–109, 133–134, 157–158, 174, 192–193, 207; know your hooks exercise, 98; life map, 52, 54; self-disclosure card shuffle, 160; stuck patterns, 86; sweet spot exercise, 72–73; values and vulnerabilities, 124; values authorship, 135; yoga practice, 70, 95, 123, 149, 165, 184, 209; your two futures meditation, 176; Zen death poem authorship, 198
deep breathing, 56
defusion, 19, 79, 95, 173
deictic framing, 173, 176
dhāranā, 43, 60
dhyāna, 107
dietary habits, 124–127
disclosure. *See* self-disclosure
discrimination task, 217
Dōgen, Eihei, 113
Downward Dog pose, 181
Drunken Table pose, 91
dry-erase board, 39

E

eating, mindful, 124–127
enlightenment, 10, 26
Escape, Avoidance, and Control Checklist, 110
exercises: ACT improv, 166; body scan, 73–75, 104; bringing your whole self to the room, 46–48; connecting to your future self, 184–186; intention-setting, 45–46, 207; know your hooks, 95–98; mindful eating, 125; placard moments, 193; saying good-bye, 209–210; self-disclosure card shuffle, 159–160; sweet spot, 70–73; three-part breathing, 158–159; values authorship, 134–135; what matters is what hurts, 104; Zen death poem authorship, 197–198. *See also* meditations; Savasana practices
extension, 34, 121
external rotation, 35

F

Facebook group for MYACT, 40–41
feeling, practice of, 180
feet, 33
femur, 32
fibula, 32
flexibility: painful experience and, 161; psychological, 2, 3, 5–7, 8
flexion, 34
floor sitting, 57
floppy mountain, 113
focus, 43
forearm, 29
forms. *See* worksheets
foundational poses, 112
freedom: pain and, 155; yoga as, 161
freestyle movement, 208
frontal plane, 34
functional analysis, 83–85
functional contextualism, 10–13, 183
functional movement, 34–35, 148
functional self-disclosure, 86, 109, 205
fusion with self-content, 22
future perspectives meditation, 174–176

G

go with it meditation, 156–157
goals: ACT and MYACT, 10; SMART, 98, 100

MORE BOOKS *from*
NEW HARBINGER PUBLICATIONS

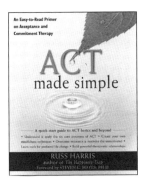

ACT MADE SIMPLE

An Easy-To-Read Primer
on Acceptance &
Commitment Therapy

978-1572247055 / US $39.95

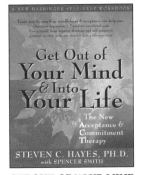

**GET OUT OF YOUR MIND
& INTO YOUR LIFE**

The New Acceptance &
Commitment Therapy

978-1572244252 / US $21.95

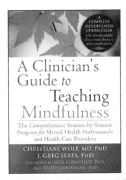

**A CLINICIAN'S GUIDE TO
TEACHING MINDFULNESS**

The Comprehensive Session-by-
Session Program for Mental Health
Professionals & Health Care Providers

978-1626251397 / US $49.95

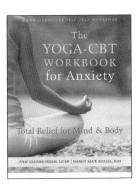

**THE YOGA-CBT
WORKBOOK
FOR ANXIETY**

Total Relief for Mind & Body

978-1626258365 / US $19.95

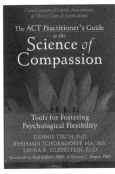

**THE ACT
PRACTITIONER'S GUIDE
TO THE SCIENCE
OF COMPASSION**

Tools for Fostering
Psychological Flexibility

978-1626250550 / US $49.95

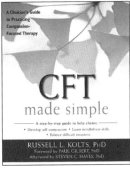

CFT MADE SIMPLE

A Clinician's Guide to Practicing
Compassion-Focused Therapy

978-1626253094 / US $49.95

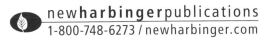

Register your **new harbinger** titles for additional benefits!

When you register your **new harbinger** title—purchased in any format, from any source—you get access to benefits like the following:

- Downloadable accessories like printable worksheets and extra content

- Instructional videos and audio files

- Information about updates, corrections, and new editions

Not every title has accessories, but we're adding new material all the time.

Access free accessories in 3 easy steps:

1. Sign in at NewHarbinger.com (or **register** to create an account).

2. Click on **register a book**. Search for your title and click the **register** button when it appears.

3. Click on the **book cover or title** to go to its details page. Click on **accessories** to view and access files.

That's all there is to it!

If you need help, visit:

NewHarbinger.com/accessories

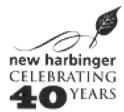

new harbinger
CELEBRATING
40 YEARS